DISCARD

D0339388

Clinical Surface Anatomy

Second Edition

Kenneth M Backhouse OBE VRD MB BS MRCS

Reader Emeritus in Applied Anatomy, University of London; Clinical Anatomist, Institute of Laryngology and Otology, University College London

Formerly Reader in Applied Anatomy, Hunterian Professor, Arris and Gale Lecturer and Examiner in Anatomy for Primary FRCS and FDS, Royal College of Surgeons of England; Member of the Occupational Therapy Board, UK; Hand Surgeon, President and Archivist, British Society for Surgery of the Hand

Ralph T Hutchings

Freelance Photographer
Formerly Chief Medical Laboratory Scientific Officer,
Royal College of Surgeons of England

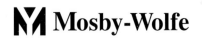

Mosby-Wolfe

571.3
B126c
1998

Copyright © 1998 Times Mirror International Publishers Limited

Published in 1998 by Mosby, an imprint of Times Mirror International Publishers Limited

Printed in Spain by Grafos S.A. Arte sobre papel, Barcelona, Spain

ISBN 0 7234 2495 0

All rights reserved. No part of this publication may be reproduced, stored in a retrieval system, copied or transmitted, in any form or by any means, electronic, mechanical, photocopying, recording or otherwise, without written permission from the Publisher or in accordance with the provisions of the Copyright Act 1988, or under the terms of any licence permitting limited copying issued by the Copyright Licensing Agency, 33–34 Alfred Place, London, WC1E 7DP, UK.

Any person who does any unauthorised act in relation to this publication may be liable to criminal prosecution and civil claims for damages.

Permission to photocopy or reproduce solely for internal or personal use is permitted for libraries or other users registered with the Copyright Clearance Center, provided that the base fee of $4.00 per chapter plus $0.10 per page is paid directly to the Copyright Clearance Center, 21 Congress Street, Salem, MA 01970, USA. This consent does not extend to other kinds of copying, such as copying for general distribution, for advertising or promotional purposes, for creating new collected works, or for resale.

For full details of all Mosby titles, please write to Mosby International, Lynton House, 7–12 Tavistock Square, London WC1H 9LB, UK.

A CIP catalogue record for this book is available from the British Library.

Library of Congress Cataloging-in-Publication Data applied for

Project Manager:	Leslie Sinoway
Developmental Editor:	Simon Pritchard
Layout:	Tim Read
Cover design:	Ian Spick
Illustration:	Mike Saiz
Production:	Siobhán Egan
Index:	Anita Reid
Publisher:	Geoff Greenwood

Contents

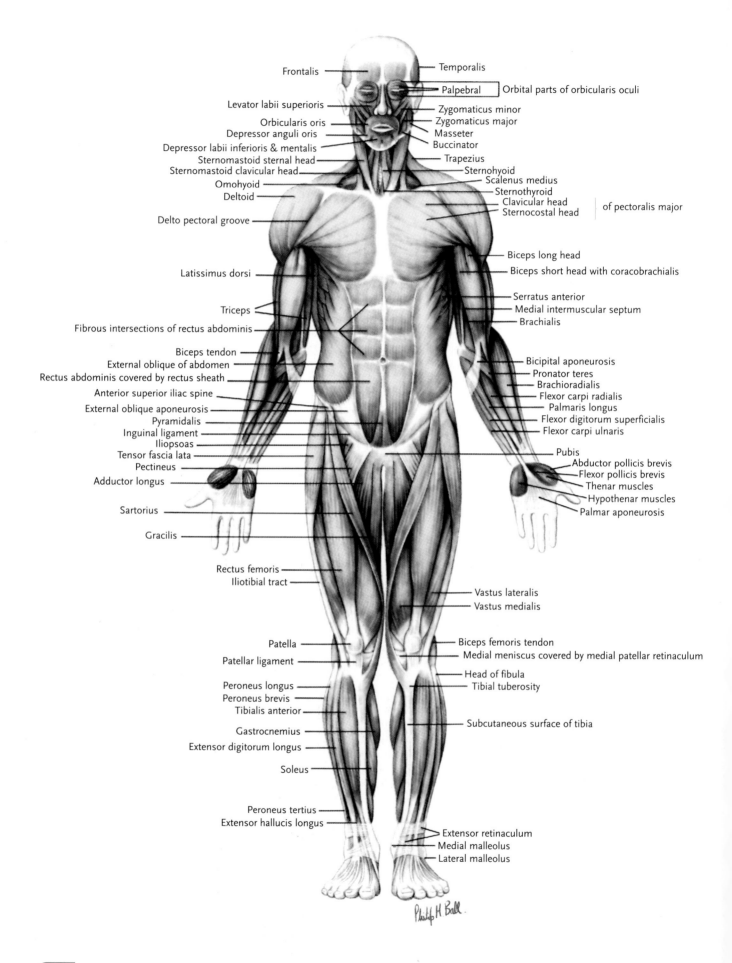

Frontalis — — Temporalis

Palpebral — Orbital parts of orbicularis oculi

Levator labii superioris — — Zygomaticus minor
Orbicularis oris — — Zygomaticus major
Depressor anguli oris — — Masseter
Depressor labii inferioris & mentalis — — Buccinator
Sternomastoid sternal head — — Trapezius
Sternomastoid clavicular head — — Sternohyoid
Omohyoid — — Scalenus medius
Deltoid — — Sternothyroid
Delto pectoral groove — — Clavicular head
— Sternocostal head

of pectoralis major

Biceps long head
Biceps short head with coracobrachialis
Latissimus dorsi —
Serratus anterior
Medial intermuscular septum
Triceps — — Brachialis
Fibrous intersections of rectus abdominis —

Biceps tendon — Bicipital aponeurosis
External oblique of abdomen — Pronator teres
Rectus abdominis covered by rectus sheath — Brachioradialis
Anterior superior iliac spine — Flexor carpi radialis
External oblique aponeurosis — Palmaris longus
Pyramidalis — Flexor digitorum superficialis
Inguinal ligament — Flexor carpi ulnaris
Iliopsoas —
Tensor fascia lata — Pubis
Pectineus — Abductor pollicis brevis
Adductor longus — Flexor pollicis brevis
— Thenar muscles
Sartorius — Hypothenar muscles
— Palmar aponeurosis

Gracilis —

Rectus femoris — Vastus lateralis
Iliotibial tract — Vastus medialis

Patella — Biceps femoris tendon
Medial meniscus covered by medial patellar retinaculum
Patellar ligament —
Head of fibula
Peroneus longus — Tibial tuberosity
Peroneus brevis —
Tibialis anterior —
Subcutaneous surface of tibia
Gastrocnemius —
Extensor digitorum longus —
Soleus —

Peroneus tertius —
Extensor hallucis longus —
Extensor retinaculum
Medial malleolus
Lateral malleolus

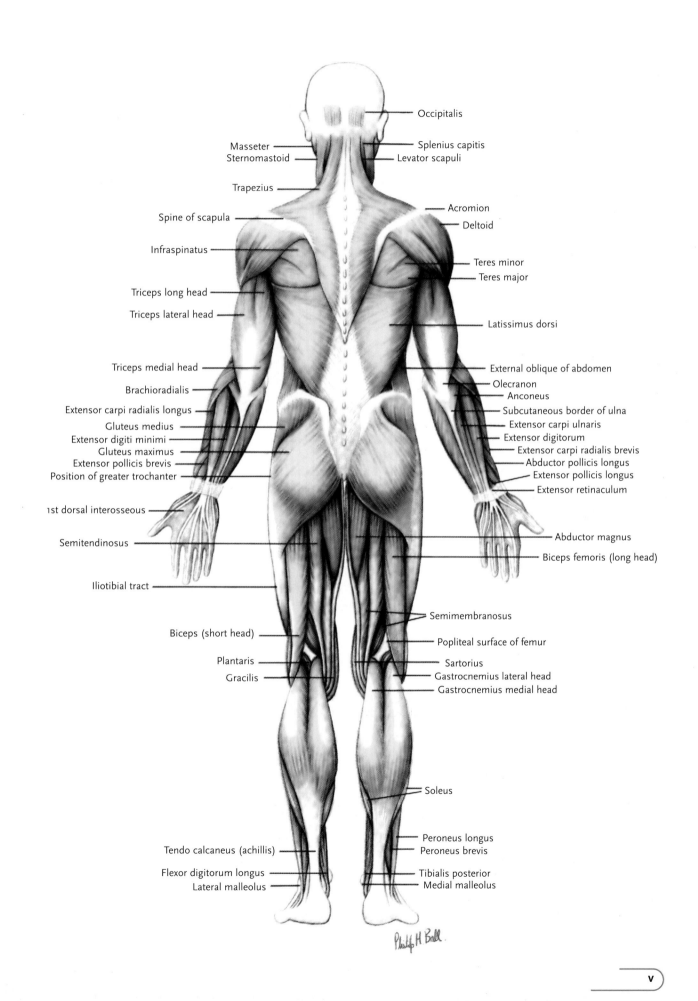

Occipitalis

Masseter
Sternomastoid

Splenius capitis
Levator scapuli

Trapezius

Spine of scapula

Acromion
Deltoid

Infraspinatus

Teres minor
Teres major

Triceps long head

Triceps lateral head

Latissimus dorsi

Triceps medial head

External oblique of abdomen

Brachioradialis

Olecranon
Anconeus

Extensor carpi radialis longus

Subcutaneous border of ulna

Gluteus medius

Extensor carpi ulnaris

Extensor digiti minimi

Extensor digitorum

Gluteus maximus

Extensor carpi radialis brevis

Extensor pollicis brevis

Abductor pollicis longus

Position of greater trochanter

Extensor pollicis longus
Extensor retinaculum

1st dorsal interosseous

Semitendinosus

Abductor magnus

Biceps femoris (long head)

Iliotibial tract

Semimembranosus

Biceps (short head)

Popliteal surface of femur

Plantaris

Sartorius

Gracilis

Gastrocnemius lateral head
Gastrocnemius medial head

Soleus

Peroneus longus
Peroneus brevis

Tendo calcaneus (achillis)

Flexor digitorum longus
Lateral malleolus

Tibialis posterior
Medial malleolus

Preface

The learning of anatomy is often considered to be primarily one of acquiring an assemblage of facts on effectively inanimate building blocks of the body—a morphological exercise. But basic structural anatomy is of little value unless it can be seen to exist and function in the living person; the anatomy must live, move, grow, age and exhibit all the genetic and developmental variations evident in the community as well as the changes consequent upon physical activity or disease. The physician, surgeon, therapist, nurse, physical educator and artist must look at the skin-covered individual and visualize what lies and functions beneath that skin; this is the primary approach to the clinical assessment of normal function and any variation from that normality, be it from injury or disease.

Many structures can be seen from their surface contours and appearance: bony points, superficial muscles, tendons, veins. For deeper structures, their surface positions need to be known from whence their functions can be assessed clinically. The normal functioning of muscles and the nervous control of the body can be examined from the surface; where pathology is suspected, a knowledge of how to test for that normality or otherwise is vital.

A thorough knowledge of surface anatomy is thus essential to the diagnosis and management of patients. Physical and clinical examination, the planning of surgical approaches, the application of regional anaesthesia, the various aspects of physical therapy all depend upon the ability to assess what lies and functions beneath the skin— simply by observing, touching and manipulating surface features.

It has been fashionable, particularly among some physicians, to claim that they have forgotten most of their anatomy and don't miss it. They dismiss lifeless morphology, their considerable knowledge of living anatomy being seen simply as an integral part of their clinical expertise. In that light, we offer this book as a basic contribution to clinical medicine.

For this second edition, we have completely rewritten the text and reduced the number of illustrations to produce, we hope, a book that is more accessible, more focused—and more affordable—than its predecessor, and one that places even greater emphasis on clinical relevance. Many of the original photographs have been replaced by new material, and a less obtrusive, more informative style of illustration has been adopted to complement the photographic material.

In photographing surface details it is always tempting to use dramatic lighting techniques and models with highly developed muscles. We continue to avoid both—the aim being to produce a good pictorial representation of the type of people a practitioner is likely to meet in everyday practice.

Clinical Surface Anatomy is designed primarily for medical and paramedical personnel. Nevertheless, it is hoped that in view of its strong emphasis on kinesiology it will be of particular value to physical educators, teachers of dance, etc. as well as a useful life study for artists.

Kenneth M Backhouse, May 1997

Chapter 1

Introduction

THE SKIN

Observation and examination of the body must begin with the skin or, in the orifices, the mucous membranes. Many disease processes affect the skin, both directly and indirectly, and its examination is of major clinical importance. The clinician also needs to be able to identify and locate underlying structures and assess their size and function from the surface.

The body must have total skin cover. A major part of a plastic surgeon's work is to replace skin after loss, using skin grafts or flaps, to give full protective covering to the body.

Skin contains the receptive components of surface sensation, i.e. **exteroceptive sensibility**, which are linked by sensory nerve paths to the brain. This is especially important in certain parts of the body. The palms of the hands are hairless and are specialised to receive very fine sensory stimuli (**epicritic sensibility**). The routine clinical testing of skin sensation is the sensibility to **pinprick and fine touch** (e.g. with cotton wool), on occasions supplemented by **temperature**. In the hand **epicritic sensibility** may be tested by the closeness of **two-point discrimination** and by the ability to identify a variety of textures, e.g. silk, wool, sandpaper, wood.

The **character of the skin** varies enormously over the body. The difference is obvious at the lips, where the relatively thinly keratinised vermilion region changes to the much thicker hairy skin of the face and the mucous membrane of the mouth. The skin on the flexor surfaces of the body is thin and much more sensitive than the thicker skin over the dorsum, with that over the back being especially thick. There are ethnic variations—not only in colour but also in other characteristics—of skin and hair.

The skin in youth adjusts to body movement by its **intrinsic elasticity**. With ageing, elasticity is lost (as in other tissues of the body); the skin becomes lined and sags, recovering poorly after deformation (**Figures 1 and 2**).

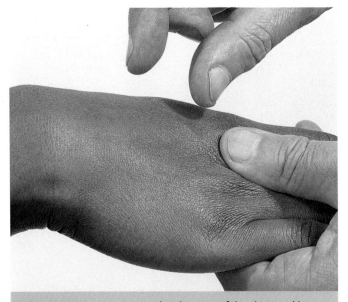

Figure 1 In a young person, the elasticity of the skin quickly returns it to its natural shape after being deformed – as when pinched.

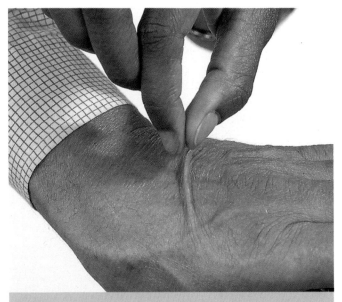

Figure 2 In an older person, the skin is slow to return to its natural shape after being pinched because of loss of elasticity.

In certain places the skin must be bound down to the underlying deep fascia, as at the **flexion creases**, to prevent movement being impaired by uncontrolled skin and subcutaneous fat.

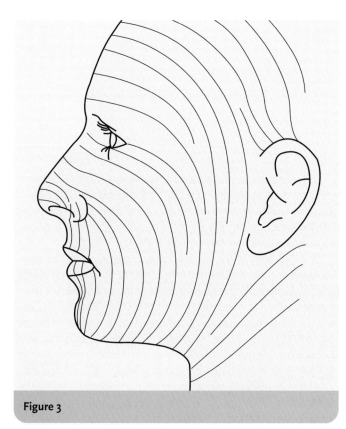

Figure 3

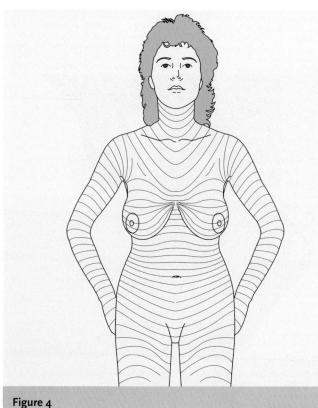

Figure 4

The skin is subject to internal stresses, which vary with site. Langer showed these to be present even in a cadaver, from which he produced his stress lines. However, Langer's lines do not always correspond with the stress lines in life; hence the term **resting stress lines (RSLs)** is now used clinically to describe stress lines in the living skin with the region at rest (**Figures 3 and 4**). Knowledge of skin stresses is important in surgery. Wounds under minimal stress (i.e. along RSLs) heal with minimal scar formation, whereas wounds across these lines and under stress heal with greater scar (fibrous tissue) formation and risk of subsequent scar contraction. The term **resting** is important. For instance, at the flexor aspect of the elbow, the RSLs follow the creases (as in most other parts of the body), i.e. here running transversely. However, if the arm is fully extended, longitudinal stresses are imparted; hence wounds, even along RSLs, should be set for repair with the skin in a resting position where possible.

In certain areas—the face and neck and the ulnar heel of the hand—striated muscle runs directly into the skin to generate movement, thus inducing **dynamic stress lines** in addition to the resting ones. In the face the so-called muscles of facial expression are inserted directly into the skin. In the region of the eye they control lid closure, while the orbital part pulls up the surrounding skin, helping shade the eyes from the sun. Note how this has generated crease lines that cross the RSLs (**Figure 5**), accentuated here by sun-browning of the surrounding skin. In other areas, e.g. the scrotum in the male and the nipples in both sexes, highly specialised involuntary muscle induces skin contraction in response to cold and other stimuli.

Hair is present over all of the body (**Figure 6**), except for such special sensory zones as the palms of the hands, soles of the feet, and lips. In the scalp, in particular, the hair shows considerable variations in structure and colour, great care often being taken over its appearance (**Figure 7**).

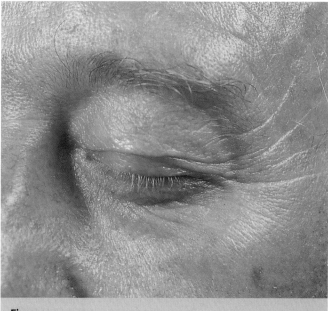

Figure 5

Baldness is common in males but in females is often of pathological significance. Natural baldness, as well as the degree of body hairiness, is both sex-linked and familial.

With sexual maturity, characteristic **body hair patterns** develop (though with genetic variation) in the axilla and the pubic region of both sexes. In females the pubic hair tends to be limited to the mons pubis (veneris) and a little on the labia majora (**Figure 8**). In males the hair tends to extend up to the umbilicus and, in more hairy individuals, may continue over the upper abdomen, increasing in amount over the chest (**Figure 9**). The face also becomes hairy (bearded) in males, though with considerable racial variation. Whereas a male may lose hair on his head, that on his body may increase with age; the ears may become hairy and the eyebrows more shaggy.

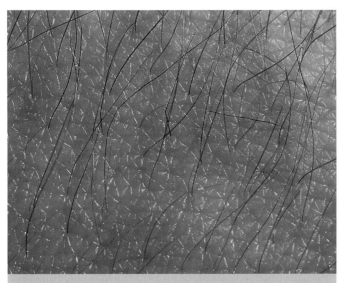

Figure 6 A magnified view of the skin on the back of a male forearm, showing the pits or follicles from which the hair grows and into which the sebaceous glands open, as well as the other openings of sebaceous and sweat glands.

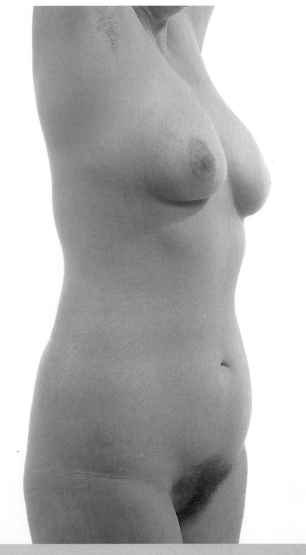

Figure 8

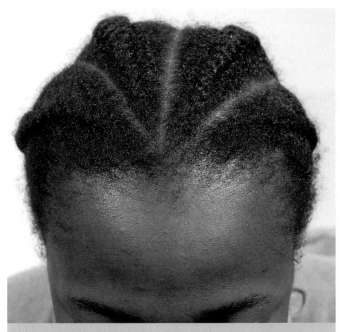

Figure 7 A form of hairdressing ideally suited to the short-growing curly negroid hair.

SURFACE CONTOURS

Sex hormones determine male and female characteristics, most obviously in the genitalia and associated sexual structures. Males tend to have a heavier build, with more bulky bone and muscle structure, though physical usage is also very important. Whereas males tend to have a more dynamic appearance, with muscle contours showing through the skin, subcutaneous fat in females tends to give them softer curves.

When fat is increased in amount, its pattern of deposition differs between the sexes. Fat is a feature of the female breasts; also the buttocks, lower abdomen, hips and thighs. Males tend to lay down fat more generally over the abdominal wall and in the mesenteries of the abdomen, to give a protruding 'corporation', though this is not the usual feature of a fit young man (**Figure 9**).

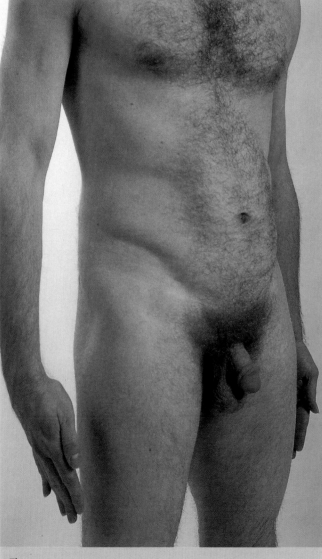

Figure 9

BONE AND MUSCLE

Much of the surface contour of the body is created by the bony skeleton and its controlling muscles. Of the axial skeleton, the skull, part of the rib cage, and the vertebral spines are readily palpable. The pelvis is hidden except for certain prominent features. Certain limb bones run subcutaneously or have palpable subcutaneous features, but otherwise are masked by muscles. Some individual muscles may be obvious from the surface, particularly in a muscular person. Some people practise forms of muscle development, such as repeated **isometric** exercising of individual muscles, that give both bulk and isolation of muscle control. This can facilitate examination. However, for most of the population, including even the athletically fit, examination may be less easy. Hard training in most physical activities, which predominantly involve **isotonic** activity, usually leads to strong but not bulky muscles. Many outstanding athletes are remarkably slim. Surface examination of individual muscles (and their nerve supply), therefore, may depend upon clinical analysis of their functions.

Muscles are elastic structures exhibiting such elastic pull as is commensurate with their size, assuming they have normal innervation. The normal state of resting muscle is termed **tone** (tonus). It is important for anyone examining muscle to be aware how normal muscle feels from the surface.

Few people can produce isolated activity in individual muscles. Examination of muscles for their individual actions, and hence the normality of their nerve supply, must often be linked with movement of a muscle group as a whole and the activity (or lack of it) of the individual muscle assessed from this. It may be necessary to compare one side with the other, particularly where action of the muscle is not readily observable from the surface.

Although a muscle may be innervated by a single nerve, it is rare for that nerve to come from a single nerve root. A muscle, therefore, may suffer from total denervation if the nerve is lost, or partial denervation if there is a root deficiency.

PROPORTIONS OF THE BODY

The proportions of the body vary enormously as it grows. In the antenatal period the nervous system must develop almost completely, in anticipation of free living, postnatal neuronal growth being mostly in length. Myelination of the nerves continues over the first $1^{1}/_{2}$–2 years, by which time the cranial cavity will approach adult size, the major growth in the skull thereafter being bony. Growth of the head continues in the facial skeleton. Meanwhile the trunk and, to a greater extent, the limbs will grow, changing the body's proportions. At birth the head is about 25% of the body length (**Figure 10**); by 2 years, 20%; and in an adult, 13%. In an adult the eyes are at the midpoint of the height of the head, but at birth they are three parts above to two below.

The midpoint of adult height is at the pubis, but at birth it is at or a little above the umbilicus. In an adult the legs contribute about half the total height; the arms from shoulder to finger tips are about 40% (**Figure 11**). The arms fully abducted to 90° span to the body height. At birth the legs contribute only 30% of the body height; the arms are, relatively, a little longer.

Facial proportions that vary from the norm are readily noticeable, though it may be less easy to perceive what is wrong. Leonardo da Vinci found analysis of facial, as well as bodily, proportions to be vital, as is true for any artist or plastic surgeon. The following details are based on Leonardo's observations.

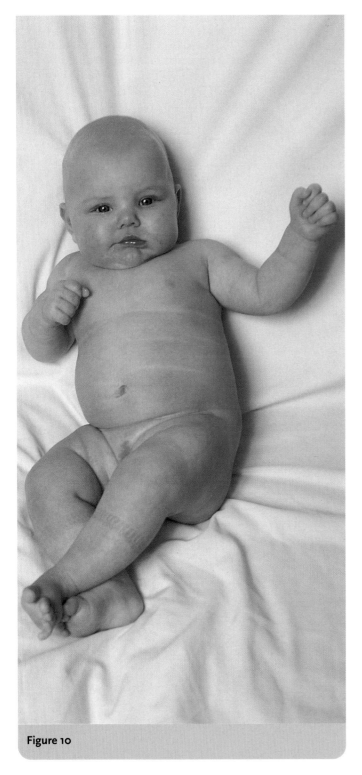

Figure 10

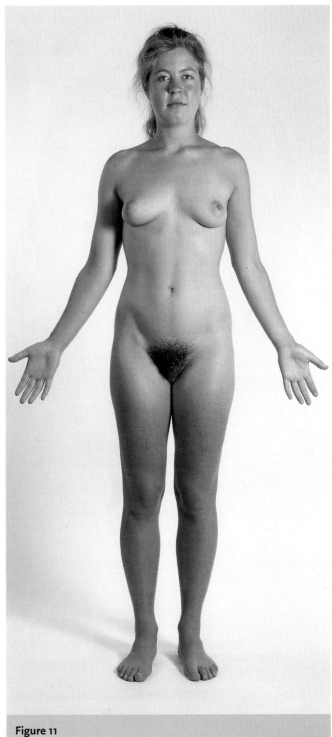

Figure 11

In an adult the eyes should be at the midpoint of the vertical height of the head (**Figure 12**). Each eye should be the same width (**Figure 13, see A**) as the distance between the eyes (**Figure 13, see B**), which should also be the width of the lower part of the nose. The width of the mouth at rest should be the same as the distance between the irises.

The upper tip of the ear should be level with the eyebrows and the glabella; the spine of the helix of the ear should be level with the root of the nose (the nasion); the tip of the nose should be level with the lobe of the ear. The crease between the lower lip and chin should be midway between the lower

aspects of the nose and chin, and level with the angle of the jaw (**Figure 12**).

Many measurements of the face follow a 'rule of thumb', i.e. the length of the thumb between its tip and metacarpophalangeal joint (**Figure 12, T**). Such is the vertical height of the ear; the distance from the ear to the lateral aspect of the eye; and from there to the midline. Similarly it gives the distance from the chin to the tip of the nose; from there to the glabella or eyebrows; and from there to the hair line. The lobe of the ear to the angle of the jaw is about $\frac{1}{2}$ thumb length, as is the width of the ear.

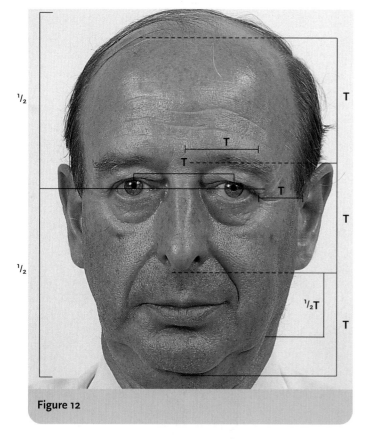

Figure 12

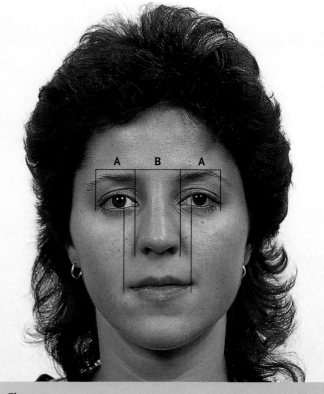

Figure 13

Chapter 2

The head

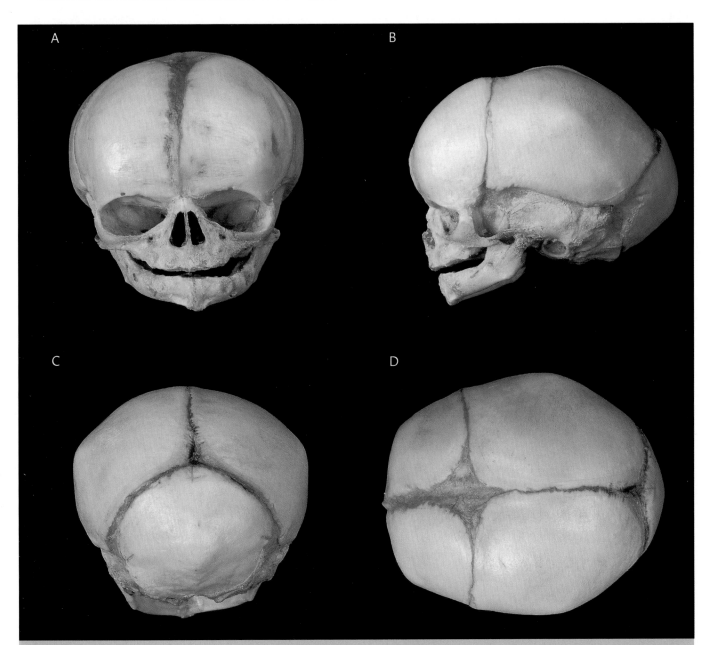

A

B

C

D

Figure 14A–D The state of ossification of the bones of the skull, as well as the form of the facial skeleton, can be seen in the four views of a skull of a newborn baby.

A = anterior
B = lateral
C = posterior
D = superior

EXAMINATION OF BONY POINTS

The major bony features of the face and head are relatively easy to examine in the normal state, but often less so through injured, swollen tissue.

The dome-like vault of the skull is flattened in the parietal region. At birth the vault is made of thin bone, joined by membranous tissue at the fontanelles (**Figure 14**). Two fontanelles are easy to feel and may bulge when the baby cries. The diamond-shaped **anterior fontanelle** is at the junction of the two parietal bones and the two frontal bones, at this stage being separated by the metopic suture (**Figure 15**). The **posterior fontanelle**, lying between the parietal and occipital bones, is triangular. The fontanelles and the metopic suture should be closed by 2 years, though the suture occasionally persists throughout life. Two lateral fontanelles are present on each side; the anterior is covered by temporalis and is impalpable, but the posterior, at the junction of the temporal, parietal and occipital bones, can usually be felt.

The **orbital margins** are readily palpable (**Figures 16 and 18, see 11**). Discontinuity of the inferior margin due to fracture can usually be felt unless the tissues are grossly swollen. NB The two sides should always be compared. The **infraorbital foramen** should be palpable midway between the nasal alar and the outer canthus of the eye, where pressure sensation on the nerve may be produced (**Figure 18, see 10**).

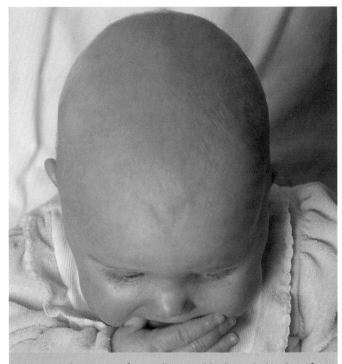

Figure 15 The anterior fontanelle is visible through the skin of this 5-month-old baby.

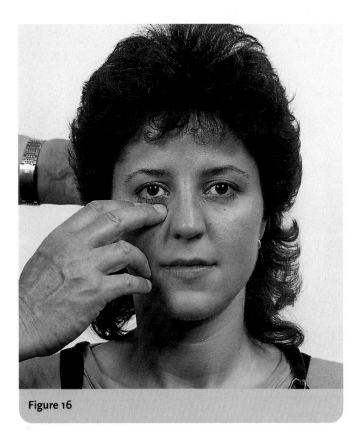

Figure 16

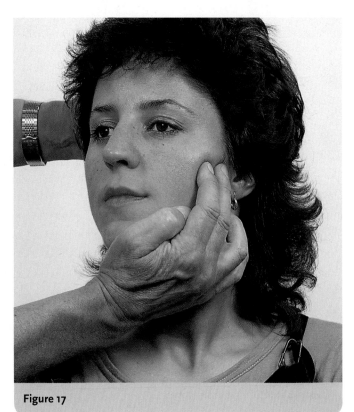

Figure 17

The **frontozygomatic suture** may be felt below the lateral tip of the eyebrow (**Figure 18, see 7 and Figure 19, see 8**). Superiorly, the **supraorbital foramen** (or **notch**) is palpable about 2.5 cm lateral to the midline (**Figure 18, see 6**) (or, take three of the patient's fingers, place the first in the midline, and the third will overlie the foramen). The **zygomatic arch** is readily palpable from below (**Figures 17 and 18, see 8**). Posteriorly it is level with the tragus, but is lower nearer the nose. The upper edge is camouflaged by the attached, tense temporal fascia. Behind the ear is the prominent **mastoid process** with its contained mastoid air cells, linked through the mastoid antrum with the middle ear (**Figure 19, see 2**).

The lower border of the **mandible** is readily palpable, as is the angle (**Figure 19, see 23 and 25**). The parotid gland overlaps all except the lowest 2.5 cm of the ramus, masking the bony details up to its head. Anteriorly, the **mental protuberance** produces a sloping shelf between the chin and anterior margin of the alveolus (**Figure 18, see 19**). Examination of the mandible must always include the **teeth and bite**. Anteriorly, the spade-like upper incisors should overlap the narrower, lower ones (**Figure 18, see 14 and 15**). Laterally, the upper outer (buccal) cusps of the premolar and molar teeth should overlap those of the lower ones (**Figure 19, see 17–21, and Figure 22**).

THE TEMPOROMANDIBULAR JOINT

This is not a true hinge joint. The head of the mandible, a transversely running cylinder (**Figure 19, see 5**), sits at rest in the articular fossa of the temporal bone, the joint cavity being divided into two by the **articular disc**. The lateral end of the head can be felt immediately in front of the tragus of the ear, below the root of the zygoma; but, as the jaw is opened, it is carried forwards onto the promontory and may be seen or felt as a slight swelling below the zygomatic arch (**Figure 23**). As the jaw is closed, the head returns to the fossa. Ideally, the joint and its controlling muscles should be examined from behind (**Figure 24**).

The temporomandibular joint normally bears little load on its joint surfaces, even in a powerful bite. The mandible is normally carried under the precisely balanced control of its muscles, allowing the whole system to be readjusted to dental change. This fine neuromuscular balance may result in major problems in bite occurring from what would appear to be minor pathology.

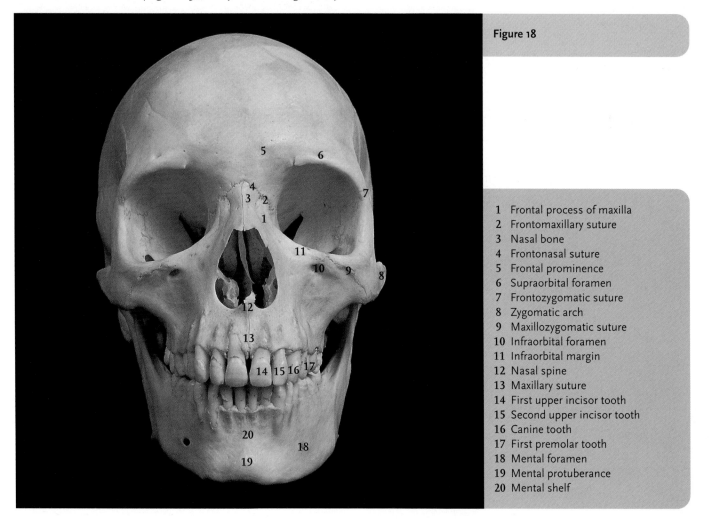

Figure 18

1 Frontal process of maxilla
2 Frontomaxillary suture
3 Nasal bone
4 Frontonasal suture
5 Frontal prominence
6 Supraorbital foramen
7 Frontozygomatic suture
8 Zygomatic arch
9 Maxillozygomatic suture
10 Infraorbital foramen
11 Infraorbital margin
12 Nasal spine
13 Maxillary suture
14 First upper incisor tooth
15 Second upper incisor tooth
16 Canine tooth
17 First premolar tooth
18 Mental foramen
19 Mental protuberance
20 Mental shelf

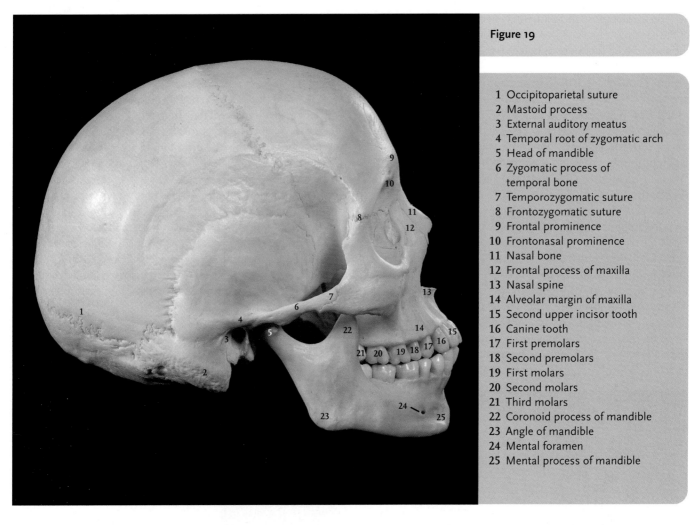

Figure 19

1 Occipitoparietal suture
2 Mastoid process
3 External auditory meatus
4 Temporal root of zygomatic arch
5 Head of mandible
6 Zygomatic process of temporal bone
7 Temporozygomatic suture
8 Frontozygomatic suture
9 Frontal prominence
10 Frontonasal prominence
11 Nasal bone
12 Frontal process of maxilla
13 Nasal spine
14 Alveolar margin of maxilla
15 Second upper incisor tooth
16 Canine tooth
17 First premolars
18 Second premolars
19 First molars
20 Second molars
21 Third molars
22 Coronoid process of mandible
23 Angle of mandible
24 Mental foramen
25 Mental process of mandible

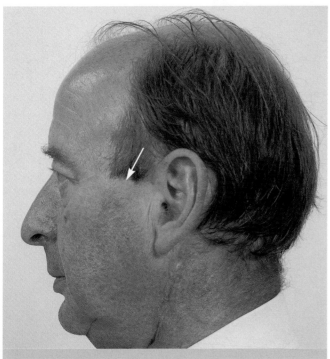

Figure 20 Surface projection of the pituitary fossa.

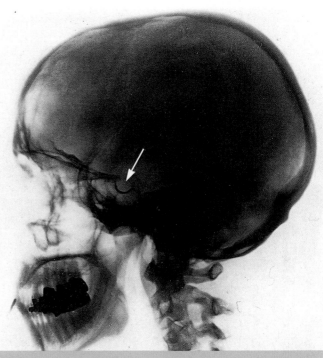

Figure 21 Radiograph of the pituitary fossa.

MUSCLES OF MASTICATION

It is usual to describe four muscles of mastication, all supplied by the **mandibular division of the trigeminal nerve**: temporalis, masseter, medial pterygoid and lateral pterygoid. However, to these should be added the muscles below and opening the mandible, so producing its balanced control. Two

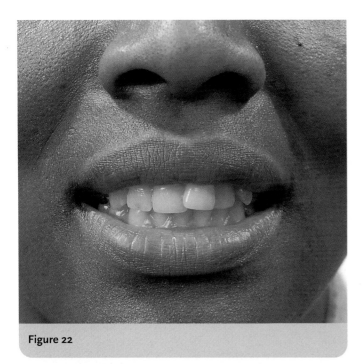

Figure 22

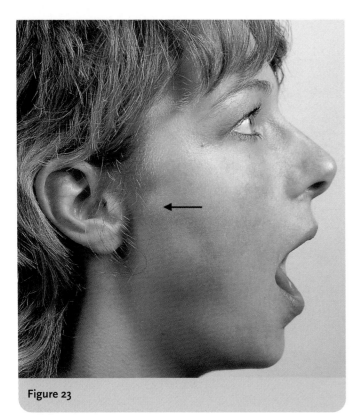

Figure 23

of these, mylohyoid and the anterior belly of the digastric, are also supplied by the mandibular nerve, through the mylohyoid branch of the inferior alveolar nerve.

The first three muscles close the jaw and, most importantly, bring its head back to the fossa. The **lateral pterygoid** assists in opening the jaw by pulling the head of the mandible forwards as the inframandibular muscles pull the jaw downwards.

The two pterygoid muscles lie deeply and so are not as readily available for direct palpation on activation as are the others (**Figure 24**). **Temporalis** originates from the side of the head over the temporal bone (i.e. above the zygomatic arch) and runs down deep to the arch, into the tip and all the anterior border of the coronoid process. It is a wide, fan-shaped muscle whose posterior fibres run forwards and retract the head of the mandible, while the anterior fibres, running vertically, pull the mandible up into a bite. From a widely open jaw, the posterior fibres can be felt acting initially to retract the head, the more anterior fibres coming progressively into action with closure. **Masseter**, below the zygoma, has obliquely running, superficial fibres that pull the angle of the mandible forwards (operating with the posterior fibres of temporalis to reposition the head) before the deeper, vertical fibres pull the mandible up into a bite. The superficial and deep heads of **medial pterygoid** act similarly to the equivalent parts of the masseter.

Activity in the **inframandibular muscles**, in both opening the jaw (particularly against resistance) and swallowing, is readily evident to palpation. In the former activity they pull the mandible down towards the hyoid; in the latter they pull up the hyoid to form a firm base for the floor of the mouth and tongue.

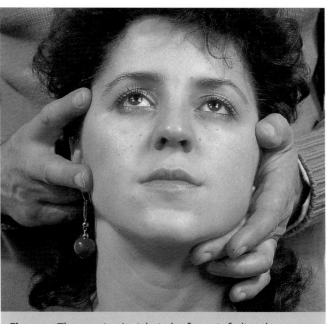

Figure 24 The examiner's right index finger is feeling the contraction of temporalis, with the middle finger that of masseter. The left middle finger feels the activity in the submandibular muscles.

THE NOSE

Both bone and cartilage support the nose. Superiorly, the **two nasal bones** each articulate laterally with the frontal process of the maxilla and above with the frontal bone, which also gives support beneath, together with the bony septum. Below, two **lateral cartilages** are effectively fused along the bridge to the septal cartilage by the perichondrium to give a strong T section. **Alar cartilages** support the nostrils (**Figure 25**).

The nose should be examined from above for symmetry, from the side and from below, as well as internally. The sharp margins of the nasal bones are obvious, overlapping the

1 Nasal bone
2 Lateral cartilage underlying nasal bone
3 Lateral cartilage
4 Membranous triangle
5 Alar cartilage—lateral crus
6 Alar cartilage—medial crus

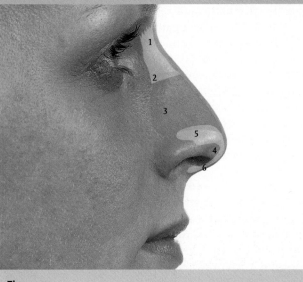

Figure 25

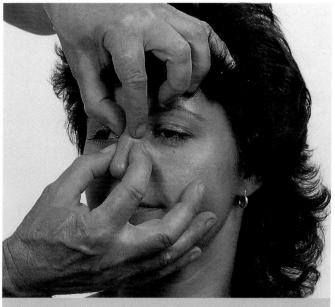

Figure 26

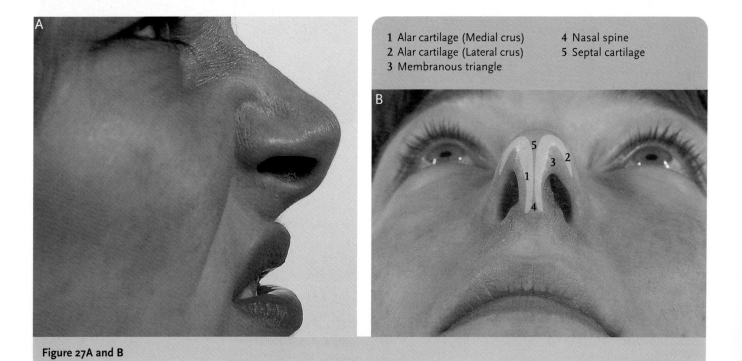

1 Alar cartilage (Medial crus)   4 Nasal spine
2 Alar cartilage (Lateral crus)   5 Septal cartilage
3 Membranous triangle

Figure 27A and B

lateral cartilages, which run beneath (**Figure 26**). Below, the lateral cartilages are overlapped by the alar cartilages, which allows their lower margins to be pulled in (**Figure 27A**) to form the so-called **nasal valves**. These valves help to spread the airflow through the nose. Each alar cartilage curves around a nostril, having a medial (septal) and a lateral crus. The two medial crura support the **columella**. They lie close together and are attached loosely to the lower end of the septal cartilage. Being quite mobile, they can be moved across to show the sharp edge of the **septal cartilage** and give easy access to it for septal surgery (**Figure 28**). At the tip of the nose the alar cartilages separate to their lateral crura. These do not follow the edge of the nostril but sweep a little upwards, leaving a membranous triangle, easily seen in **Figure 27B**. The outermost edge of the nostril is supported by a pad of fibrous material with small pieces of cartilage.

The **nasal sinuses** are of major clinical importance. Their surface projection can only be approximate in view of the variations in size (**Figure 29**). This is evident in the **frontal sinuses**, which may be little more than small upward extensions, from the anterior ethmoidal cells into the frontal bone (after the cranial bones have thickened) to major expansions upwards and over the orbits. Particularly important is the surface reference of pain from the sinuses. Pain from a **frontal sinus**, innervated by the supraorbital nerve, is referred to the overlying skin supplied by the same nerve. The **ethmoidal cells** lying between the nose and orbit are mainly supplied by branches of the nasociliary nerve (VI), while posterior cells, together with the **sphenoid sinus**, receive branches from the pterygopalatine ganglion (V2). Pain from both cells and sinus can be referred towards the inner aspect of the eye. However, pain from these being largely around the inner aspect of the eye, may also be confusing. Pain from the posterior region

can be transmitted to the ear and mastoid region. The **maxillary antrum** fills the maxilla, with only very thin bone separating it from the orbit (so allowing the globe to drop in facial fractures). It can also extend down into the alveolar region around the roots of the posterior teeth, as far forwards as the premolars. It is innervated by the infraorbital nerve (as are the upper teeth), with pain referred to the overlying cheek and often to the upper teeth.

THE EYE

This is a globe, supported and controlled by ligaments and muscles within the bony socket. The **cornea** is the central transparent part of the otherwise white opaque **sclera** of the globe. Behind the periphery of the cornea, and in front of the focusing lens, is the circular **iris**, a variously coloured diaphragm, which expands and contracts due to activity of its intrinsic muscles to control the amount of light entering the eye: the pupil is small in bright light, wider in poor light.

The **lids** protect the globe and fit closely, except at the medial commissure, where a small space forms the **lachrymal lake**. Here, the **lachrymal caruncle** is obvious, as is the **plica semilunaris** (**Figure 30**). The **lachrymal gland** lies beneath the lateral

1 Frontal sinus (small)
2 Frontal sinus (large)
3 Frontal sinus (sensory reference area)
4 Sphenoidal sinus
5 Ethmoidal sinuses (with reference area, green)
6 Maxillary antrum
7 Maxillary reference area to skin
8 Maxillary reference area to teeth

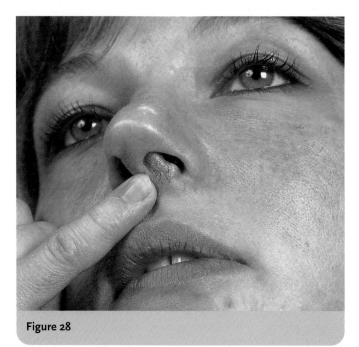

Figure 28

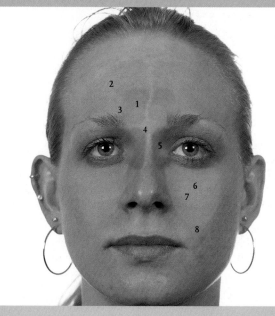

Figure 29 Surface projection of sinuses and sensory areas.

side of the upper lid. **Puncta** at the medial aspect of each lid carry tears to drain through the lachrymal sac and nasolachrymal duct into the inferior meatus of the nose.

The lids are supported by fibrocartilaginous **tarsal plates**, which are attached medially to the bone by a strong **medial palpebral ligament**. This ligament not only fixes the medial part of the lids but also overlies the lachrymal sac. The superior tarsal plate extends through the lid and must be bent in order for the upper lid to be retracted (**Figure 31**), unlike the lower lid with a narrow plate (**Figure 32**).

The lids are lined by a thin serous membrane, the **conjunctiva**, which is continuous with the skin at the lid edge and firmly adherent to the tarsi on their global surface. On the upper lid the conjunctiva extends as far as the orbital margin; on the lower lid it extends almost as far, before being reflected onto the eyeball, the reflection being known as the **fornix**. Laterally, the fornix extends to the equator of the globe, but medially it is limited by the **lachrymal caruncle** and the **plica semilunaris**. Where the conjunctiva is reflected onto the globe it lies loosely, but at about 3 mm from the cornea it becomes more closely related—but still separable surgically—up to the cornea. It fuses with the cornea at the **conjunctival annulus**, some 1 mm over the edge from the **corneal limbus**. The rich vascularity of the lid and sclera is evident (**Figure 32**), with the vessels running between the conjunctiva and sclera; however, these cease at the limbus, leaving the **cornea avascular**. On retracting the lower lid, the appearance of the blood vessels through the transparent conjunctiva can permit, with experience, a reasonable clinical **assessment of haemoglobin levels**.

The posterior parts of the eye are lined by the pigmented **retina** and the vascular **choroid**, observable by ophthalmoscopy. The retina is continued over the surface of the ciliary body and thence onto the posterior surface of the iris. It is the retinal pigment that gives the **basic blue colour to the iris** (**Figure 32**), additional colour being the result of pigment laid down in its anterior layers. In the iris an outer anastomotic ring of blood vessels sends radial branches inwards to another anastomosis in the free margin. The architecture can be seen when not overlaid with pigment (**Figure 32**).

1 Medial commissure of lids
2 Lachrymal caruncle
3 Plica semilunaris
4 Pupil
5 Iris
6 Sclera (covered by conjunctiva)
7 Openings of glands on lid margins
8 Eyelashes

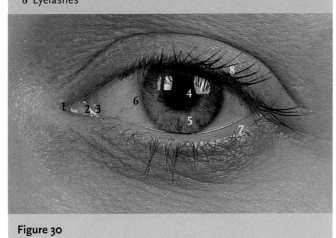

Figure 30

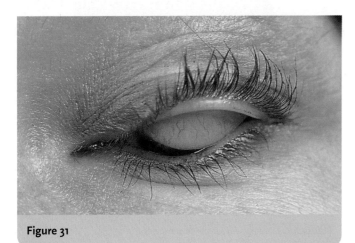

Figure 31

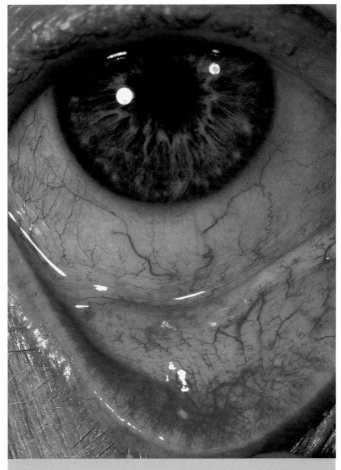

Figure 32

INTRINSIC MUSCLES OF THE EYE

These control the lens for focus (accommodation) and, in the iris, control light intensity. The lens, lying behind the iris, is controlled by ciliary muscles that act against the elasticity of the lens to focus incident light onto the retina. The effectiveness of the system can be shown by examining long and short vision. The muscular activity of the iris is more obvious. Circular muscle, controlled by the parasympathetic nerves, constricts the pupil in response to bright light (**Figure 33A**); in lower light intensities the pupil dilates under sympathetic control (**Figure 33B**).

THE EXTRAOCULAR MUSCLES

Six extraocular muscles are responsible for both balanced positioning of the eye in the socket and control of movement. The **lateral rectus** runs in the axis of the globe and pulls it laterally (abduction), whereas the **medial rectus** has the opposite effect (adduction). The other four muscles run, two above and two below, from a position medial to the axis of the globe and hence have a more complicated function. Thus, the **superior rectus** elevates and adducts, whereas the **inferior rectus** depresses and adducts. The **superior oblique** depresses and abducts, whereas the **inferior oblique** elevates and abducts.

Loss of the pull of a muscle, due to damage to either the muscle or its nerve supply, will lead to overaction of its antagonist, producing diplopia (double vision) and strabismus (squint). Thus, loss of the **lateral rectus or its nerve, the abducent**, leads to internal strabismus due to uncontrolled pull of the medial rectus. Loss of the **superior oblique (trochlear nerve)** could mean loss of downward and outward pull; however, as the other muscles can usually give some semblance of balance, the loss may only become obvious when tired. Nevertheless, as the oblique muscles also induce rotation in the globe, the superior oblique, because of the line of the inferior rectus, is important in depression in adduction. Hence, examination for a trochlear nerve lesion—albeit unusual alone—is tested for by nasal depression of the globe. The remaining muscles are supplied by the **oculomotor nerve**. Loss of this nerve leaves only the two aforesaid muscles to set the eye looking outwards and a little downwards. In addition, as the oculomotor nerve also supplies **levator palpebrae superioris**, there will be **ptosis** (drooping of the eyelid) and, owing to loss of its parasympathetic component, the pupil will be dilated (due to unopposed sympathetic action), with loss of light reflex and loss of accommodation and convergence.

Many minor cases of muscular imbalance pass unnoticed unless special ophthalmological tests are carried out. More gross levels can readily be observed by asking the person to hold their head still and follow a finger towards the periphery of vision (**Figures 34A–E**). Notice in vertical movement how the upper lid adjusts likewise.

In order to maintain binocular vision, the eyes only work in parallel in long-distance viewing. As the object moves closer, the eyes must converge, so that when the object is close, the eyes appear to be squinting (**Figure 34F**).

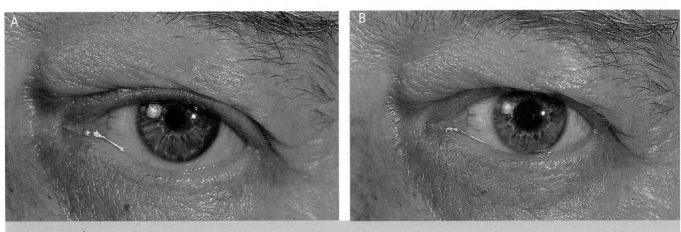

Figure 33A and B

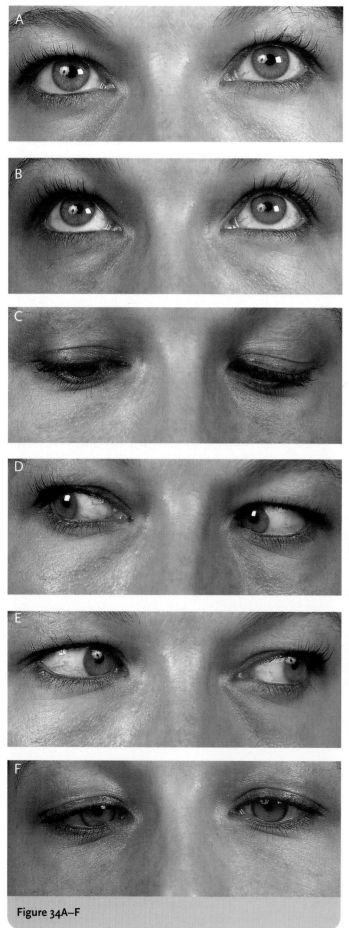

THE EXTERNAL EAR

The **auricle or pinna** is built upon a single piece of **elastic fibro-cartilage**, which shows the essential contours of the ear (**Figure 35**). Many deformities of the ear, such as 'bat-ears', arise from deformity of the cartilage, thus any surgical treatment must include the cartilage. The cartilage of the pinna is continuous with the **cartilaginous external acoustic meatus**, which in turn is joined to the margins of the bony meatus by fibrous tissue.

The **skin of the ear** is thin and bound to the underlying cartilage, particularly on the lateral (conchal) aspect, which also has numerous sebaceous glands. The **acoustic meatus** is guarded by stiff hairs, growing particularly on the tragus, anti-tragus and incisure. Hairiness often increases in older males.

The **lobule** contains no cartilage, being a variably shaped mass of fibro-fatty material.

The ear has both **external and internal muscles**, supplied by the **facial nerve**: the former able to position the pinna in relation to the head and the latter possibly varying the shape of the pinna. The external muscles produce little movement, though they have been shown, electromyographically, to react to sound stimulation.

1 Helix	8 Tragus
2 Auricular tubercle	9 Antihelix
3 Scaphoid fossa	10 Intertragic incisure
4 Triangular fossa	11 Antitragus
5 Crura of antihelix	12 Tail of helix
6 Crus of helix	13 Lobule
7 Concha	14 External acoustic meatus

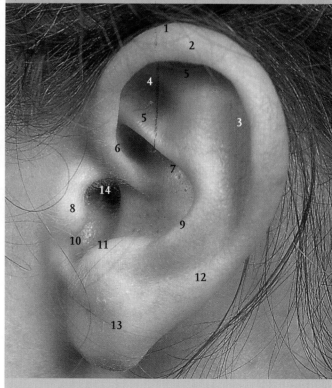

Figure 34A–F

Figure 35

The **sensory nerve supply** of the ear is complicated. C2 and C3 supply much of the surface but, as cranial nerves are also involved, the areas of supply are both variable and overlapping. The **greater auricular** nerve (C2–C3) innervates most of the cranial (posterior) surface and much of the lateral aspect of the helix, antihelix and lobule, while the **lesser occipital** supplies the upper part of the cranial surface. The **auriculotemporal** branch of the mandibular nerve supplies the tragus, crus and part of the helix. The **vagus**, with fibres from the **glosso-pharyngeal** and **facial** nerves, supplies part of the concavity of the concha, the posterior part of the external auditory meatus and the drum; a few fibres also supply a small area around the junction of the cranial surface and the mastoid process.

THE MUSCLES OF FACIAL EXPRESSION

These are muscles that are supplied by the **facial nerve** (seventh cranial) and act **directly upon the skin of the face**. Although they generate facial expression, their prime functions are controlling the eyelids, the cheeks and mouth.

Orbicularis oculi has two major and dissimilar components. The **palpebral** part, running through the lids from the thick medial palpebral ligament, is rapid-acting muscle, responsible for lid closure while maintaining the lids, and therefore the lachrymal puncta, in contact with the globe. A subunit, the **lachrymal** part, runs behind and into the lachrymal sac and, in association with lid movement, maintains the flow of tears. The **orbital** part is redder, cruder, slower-acting muscle, responsible for bunching up the periorbital tissues to protect the eye, or may be used to shade the eyes from bright light (**Figure 36A**).

Levator palpebrae superioris (oculomotor nerve), the elevator of the lid, is the antagonist of the palpebral part of orbicularis oculi, while **frontalis** acts to pull up the forehead against the orbital part (**Figure 36B**). Occipitalis, controlling the galea aponeurotica of the scalp at the back, is attached to bone (superior nuchal line), but its anterior counterpart, frontalis, intermingles with the orbital part of orbicularis oculi and is attached to the skin. Hence fluid collecting under the galea of the scalp is free to track down into the eyelids. With ageing and loss of skin elasticity the lids tend to become baggy, with an increase in soft fat, both superficial and deep to the muscle (**Figure 36**).

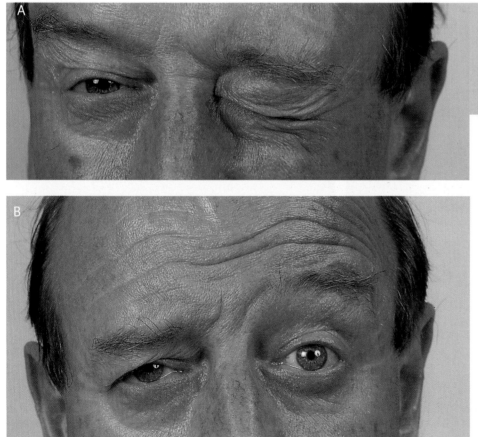

Figure 36A and B The right eye shows the orbital part of orbicularis occuli giving shading; the left, complete soft-tissue closure (**A**). The action of frontalis is seen in the left eye (B).

Buccinator controls the cheek, the muscle on each side being continuous with the superior constrictor of the pharynx through the pterygomandibular raphe. Its fibres run to the mouth to produce a smile, but essentially it holds the cheek against the teeth (**Figure 37**), preventing food collecting outside the teeth and playing an important part in dental hygiene. The buccinator muscles divide at the mouth to sweep into the lips, to form much of **orbicularis oris**, the sphincter muscle of the mouth. It is supported by small facial muscles from above and below, whose variably combined actions control lip movement.

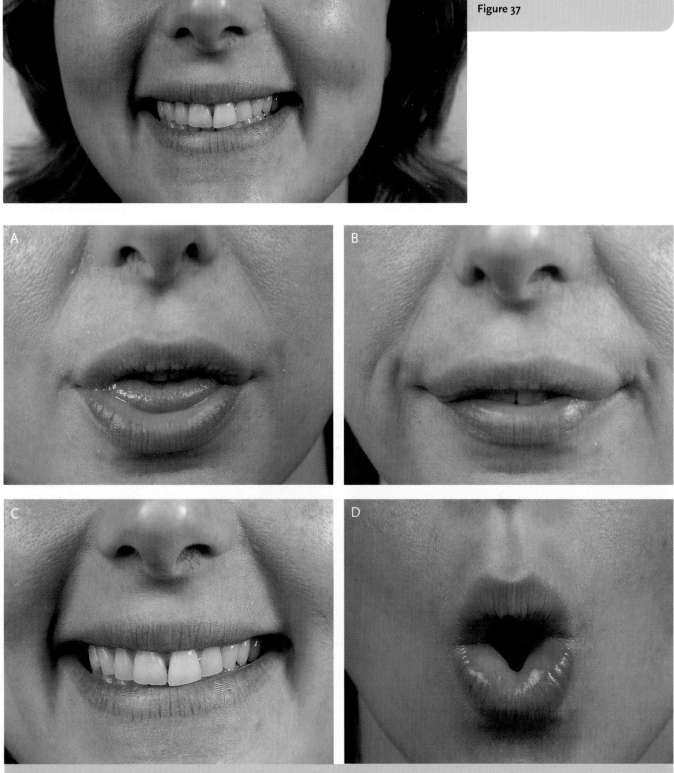

Figure 37

Figure 38A–D

FACIAL MUSCULATURE AND SPEECH

The production of sound, both volume and pitch, is primarily a laryngeal function (**phonation**). The modification of the sound into the basic components of speech (**articulation**) is supralaryngeal.

Sphincteric control of both the pharynx with the soft palate, and the palate with the tongue, are necessary to allow the explosive 'g', 'k' and 't' sounds. A juxtaposition of tongue with palate, keeping an open palatopharyngeal sphincter, is required for the sounds 's', 'n', 'ee' and 'r', which thus need fine lingual control. Apposition of tongue and teeth is required for 'th' (**Figure 38A**). Other sounds require the activity of the lips, either to produce a complete initial seal, as for 'p' and 'b', or for the lower lip to be pressed against the upper teeth, as for 'f' and 'v' (**Figure 38B**). Open lips with linguopalatal approximation are required for 'ee' and 'y' (**Figure 38C**), whereas rounded constricted lips are needed for 'o' and 'oo' (**Figure 38D**). Thus, in addition to an effective larynx, speech requires fine control of the pharynx, soft palate, tongue, cheeks and lips, with an equally effective breath control from the respiratory muscles and, particularly for maximal efficiency, the diaphragm and upper abdominal musculature.

THE CRANIAL NERVES

The cranial nerves are not all limited in their effect upon the head. Some are mixed motor and sensory, some are purely special sensory, and others also carry parasympathetic fibres.

Olfactory nerves (1) linked to the olfactory bulb are distributed to the upper part of the nasal mucosa and testing for these depends upon detection of various scents. It should be noted that taste, which is usually associated with the tongue, depends for most of its qualities upon nasal olfactory stimulation via the posterior choanae and the pharynx.

Optic nerves (2) transmit visual impulses from the retina to the brain and failure results in loss of vision. The normal neural pattern of the body is that one side is represented on the other side of the brain (excepting the cerebellum). With optic representation this pattern persists, as far as light fields are concerned, due to nasal retinal fibres crossing over at the optic chiasma (**Figure 39**). The macula, for central vision, has double representation. Note that central vision gives fine visual detail and colour perception, while the wide-ranging peripheral vision responds particularly to movement, as of the finger in Figure 39.

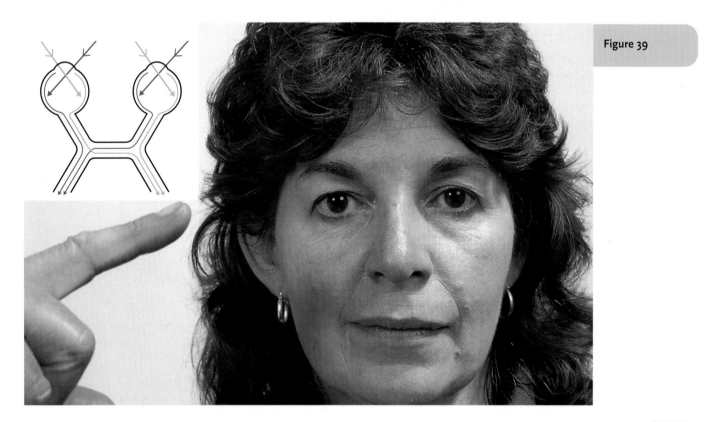

Figure 39

Oculomotor (3), trochlear (4) and abducent nerves (6) all give motor control to the extraocular muscles, whose functions and examination have been described with the eye (pages 15 and 16). The oculomotor nerve also carries parasympathetic fibres to the **intrinsic ocular muscles**, of which the pupil constrictors are the easiest for rapid examination.

The trigeminal nerve (5) has three sensory divisions (**Figure 40**), the ophthalmic, maxillary and mandibular, the last also having a motor root running with it.

The **ophthalmic division** travels through the orbit, supplying the eyeball, conjunctiva, upper lid, the skin of the forehead (supraorbital and supratrochlear nerves) up to the vertex of the scalp, the external nose and the anterior part of its internal mucosa, together with the frontal and ethmoidal sinuses.

The **maxillary division** runs into the pterygopalatine fossa from where it supplies the meninges, nasal mucosa, palate, upper teeth, maxillary sinus and the skin of the anterior part of the cheek and upper lip.

The **mandibular division** supplies skin of the temporal region, part of the ear, lateral cheek and chin, including mucosa of the cheek, the anterior $^2/_3$ of the tongue and the lower teeth.

Local regional anaesthetic blocks of these nerves or their branches are often necessary.

The main ophthalmic division is in the ophthalmological field, therefore its details are not included here.

The **supraorbital nerve** runs onto the forehead via the supraorbital notch or foramen (**Figure 41**). The **supratrochlear** lies a little medial to it, directly above the medial canthus of the eye. The supraorbital foramen is usually palpable two fingers' breadth from the midline (or, taking three of the patient's fingers and putting the first in the midline, the third will overlie the foramen).

Local anaesthetic block of these nerves may be effective for the anterior part of the scalp and forehead, but local infiltration will often be needed due to the overlap of innervation.

The main trunks of the **maxillary and mandibular nerves** lie deep; the former in the pterygopalatine fossa, anterior to the lateral pterygoid plate, and the latter at the foramen ovale, near the root of the free edge of the plate. The plate lies deep to the mandibular notch (**Figure 42**). For the maxillary nerve, the needle is inserted above the mandibular notch and below the zygomatic arch, about 1 cm anterior to the head of the mandible. On reaching the plate, the needle is directed anterosuperiorly, to enter the fissure. For the mandibular nerve, the needle is directed upwards and backwards until it just passes the edge of the plate. This region is richly vascular due to the pterygoid plexus of veins, and some local bleeding is to be expected and the patient warned. As always, care must be taken not to inject directly into a vein.

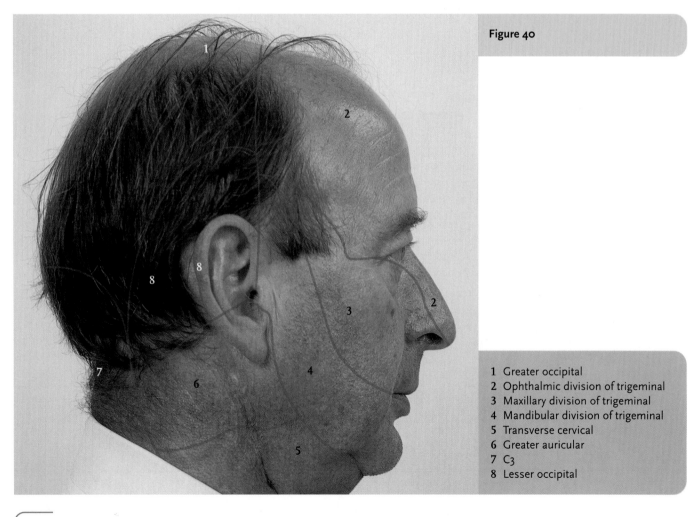

Figure 40

1 Greater occipital
2 Ophthalmic division of trigeminal
3 Maxillary division of trigeminal
4 Mandibular division of trigeminal
5 Transverse cervical
6 Greater auricular
7 C3
8 Lesser occipital

The **infraorbital nerve** may be blocked at the infraorbital foramen (**Figure 43**), palpated by placing one finger by the alar of the nose, when the adjoining finger will overlie the foramen. The foramen also lies on a line between the supraorbital and mental foramina.

Of the branches of the mandibular division, the **auriculotemporal nerve** runs behind the head of the mandible, passes through the **parotid gland** (which it supplies), to run upwards over the zygomatic arch, just behind the superficial temporal artery. As this artery can be readily palpated over the zygoma and temporal fascia (see *arteries*, page 33), the nerve's position should be easy to find.

The **lingual and inferior alveolar nerves** run together, medial to the mandible. The **lingual nerve** is accessible as it lies under the buccal mucous membrane, level with the roots of the third molar tooth, where it is also at risk in surgical removal of an impacted tooth. Although carrying sensory and taste (from the **chorda tympani**) fibres to the anterior ²⁄₃ of the tongue, its loss is rarely as severe as might be expected.

The **inferior alveolar nerve** is available to anaesthetise the mandibular teeth. The nerve enters the mandible behind the third molar tooth. With the jaw opened wide, the pterygomandibular raphe is stretched, so fixing the mucous membrane for easy entry of the needle (**Figure 44**). The needle is passed

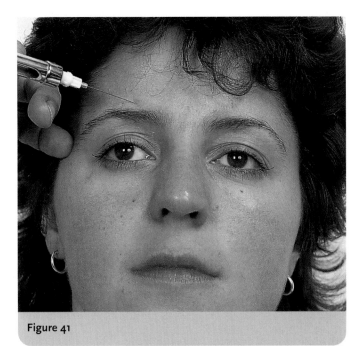

Figure 41

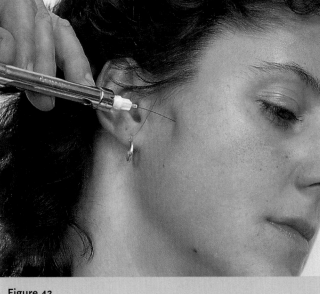

Figure 42

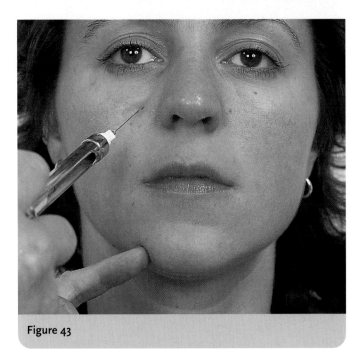

Figure 43

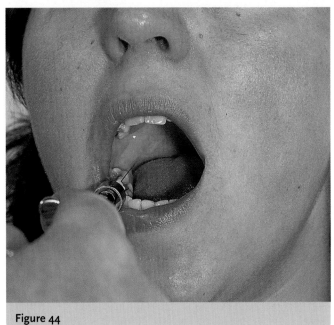

Figure 44

backwards and somewhat laterally, level with the occlusal surface of the molar teeth, running close to the bone, to the midpoint of the ramus. Sometimes, the thick tendon of temporalis muscle, at its lowest point, interferes with the needle's progress; if so, a more medial approach may be needed. As the **lingual nerve** runs close by, it is often included, anaesthetising the anterior part of the tongue as well as the expected mandibular teeth and skin of the chin. The **nerve to mylohyoid** may also be included, producing some sensation of difficulty in swallowing.

The **mental** branch of the inferior alveolar nerve leaves the mental foramen to supply the skin of the chin and lower lip. The foramen can often be felt level with the second premolar tooth and, in an adult with teeth, midway between the gingival margin and the lower border of the mandible (in a child or edentulous adult it lies higher). It is about one finger's breadth anterior to the border of the masseter and the readily palpable facial artery. (Note: the supraorbital, infraorbital and mental foramina are on a straight vertical line on the face.)

The **motor component of the mandibular nerve** has been considered in the section on mastication on page 11. The nerve also supplies **tensor tympani and tensor veli palatini**, the latter being responsible for the firm (tensor) control of the soft palate and for opening the pharyngotympanic tube to balance air pressure in the middle ear, by swallowing.

The **facial nerve (7)** carries both parasympathetic and taste fibres, but these leave the main trunk within the skull. When the nerve leaves the **stylomastoid foramen** it is, functionally, mainly motor. (Its sensory fibres are of uncertain function.) The stylomastoid foramen lies in front of the mastoid process, superficial to and a little posterior to the styloid process. The **styloid process** gives resistance if the finger is pressed between the mastoid process and the mandible and just below the external acoustic meatus. Surgically, the facial nerve can be found by dividing anterior to sternomastoid muscle at its

1 Mastoid process
2 Styloid process
3 Mandible
4 Facial nerve-posterior branches
5 Facial nerve-stylohyoid branch
6 Facial nerve-upper division
7 Facial nerve-lower division

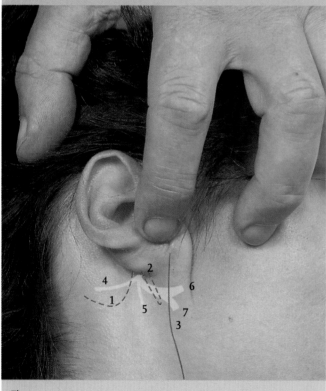

Figure 45

1 Temporal
2 Zygomatic
3 Buccal
4 Mandibular
5 Cervical

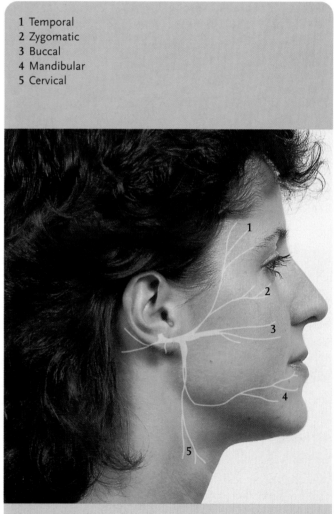

Figure 46 Facial nerve branches on the face

attachment to the mastoid process, just below the cartilaginous external auditory meatus (**Figure 45**). (The mastoid process does not develop until after the age of 2 years; until then, the facial nerve, being unprotected by bone, is vulnerable, particularly in a forceps delivery.) The nerve gives posterior branches to **occipitalis**, the **auricular muscles**, the **posterior belly of digastric and stylohyoid muscles** and then **enters the parotid gland**. Here it divides in a very variable manner. Commonly it divides first into upper and lower divisions, which further divide into five branches or sets of branches. The upper division gives **temporal** and (often multiple) **zygomatic** branches. The lower division gives the **mandibular** and **cervical** branches, while the **buccal** branch or branches come from either division or both (**Figure 46**).

The **mandibular** branch runs superficially along the lower border of the mandible before entering the face with the facial artery, at the anterior border of masseter, to supply the muscles of the lower lip. The **cervical** branch supplies platysma, the **buccal**, buccinator and orbicularis oris, the **zygomatic**, the lower parts of orbicularis oculi, nasal muscles and elevators of the upper lip, while the **temporal** supplies muscles of the forehead and the major part of orbicularis oculi. These muscles are described on pages 17 and 18.

Facial nerve loss is very unpleasant. The muscles controlling the two sides of the mouth are normally balanced. Loss on one side leads to the mouth being pulled to the normal side; this interferes with buccal function, including articulation of labial sounds. Test for this part of the nerve by asking the patient to purse their lips, blow out their cheeks and whistle. Loss of the upper branches leads to the inability to wrinkle the brow and, far more important, the loss of lid closure; the lids fall away from the globe so that the puncta are no longer in contact with the globe for the collection of tears, which pour onto the face. Partial loss is tested by forced closure of the lids.

The **vestibulocochlear nerve (8)** is the nerve responsible for hearing (from the cochlear component) and for balance (by the vestibular part). It has no extracranial course. Hearing can be tested crudely by whispering, or better by tuning fork (512 Hz). In **Weber's test** the tuning fork is activated and placed centrally over bone, such as the forehead, to check the equality of sound in each ear. In **Rinne's test** the tuning fork is set against the mastoid, and bone conduction is compared with hearing through air close to the ear, which should be better if there is no conductive hearing loss.

The **glossopharyngeal nerve (9)** contains motor, sensory and parasympathetic fibres. Sensory fibres come from the posterior third of the tongue (including taste), the tonsillar area and the oro- and laryngopharynx. Stylopharyngeus is the only muscle supplied, which, being an elevator of the pharynx and larynx, is of some importance in swallowing. Secretomotor fibres reach the parotid gland via the auriculotemporal nerve. Isolated loss of the nerve is unusual, but if it occurs, as well as loss of pain fibres, there may be slight reduction in the gag reflex from the tongue, palate and pharynx, though here there is considerable vagal overlap.

The **vagus nerve (10)** has a wide influence, including its important parasympathetic supply for the thoracic and abdominal viscera. It leaves the skull, with the glossopharyngeal and accessory nerves, via the **jugular foramen**, which lies 1 cm deeper and a few millimetres anterior to the facial nerve. This is 2 cm deep to the notch below the tragus of the ear (intertragic incisure). Then the nerve runs down the neck, along with the internal and common carotid arteries and the internal jugular vein, within the carotid sheath, to cross behind the sternoclavicular joints into the thorax (**Figure 47**).

Close to the jugular foramen the vagus is joined by the cranial part of the **accessory nerve**, the conjoined nerves supplying palatal and pharyngeal muscles through the pharyngeal branch. The vague also gives sensory supply to the epiglottis and upper larynx, and motor supply to the cricothyroid via the superior laryngeal branch, which also supplies the cricopharyngeal sphincter. The remainder of the laryngeal muscles

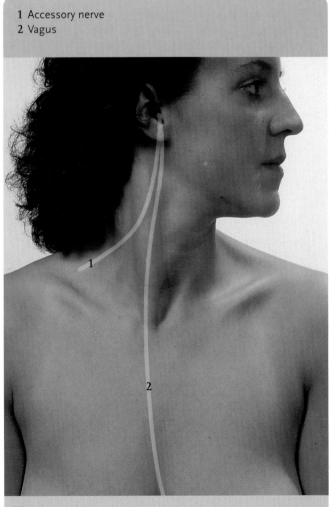

1 Accessory nerve
2 Vagus

Figure 47

and the sensory supply to the lower larynx all come from the recurrent laryngeal branch, which also supplies the upper oesophagus.

Loss of the pharyngeal branch would paralyse both the soft palate and pharynx, inducing dysphagia and, through palatal failure, a cleft-palate form of speech. Movement of the soft palate can be observed as the patient sounds 'ah' (**Figure 48**). **Paralysis of the laryngeal nerves**, particularly the recurrent, leads to dysphonia.

The **spinal accessory nerve (11)** arises from the upper five segments of the spinal cord dorsal to the motor roots, enters the cranial cavity through the foramen magnum, and joins and leaves with the cranial accessory nerve. When this joins the vagus the spinal part continues, entering the deep part of sterno-mastoid muscle, to which it gives motor innervation. Leaving about half way down the posterior border, it runs across the roof of the posterior triangle of the neck and enters trapezius about 5 cm above the clavicle, giving it a motor supply. The surface marking of the nerve can be a line drawn from below the tragus to that point on the trapezius (**Figure 47**). Action of sterno-mastoid is shown on page 29 and trapezius (and its loss) on pages 41 and 42.

The **hypoglossal nerve (12)** supplies the muscles of the tongue (except palatoglossus, responsible for the palatoglossal sphincter). If the nerve on one side is lost, that half of the tongue atrophies, and, if the tongue is protruded, it deviates to the side of the lesion.

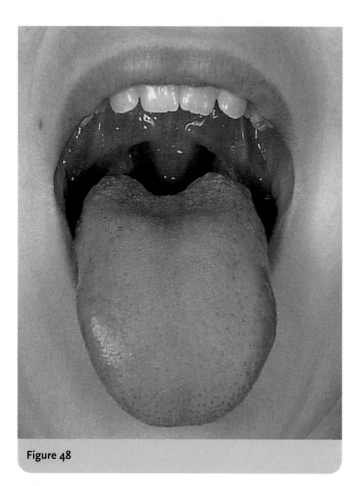

Figure 48

BLOOD SUPPLY OF THE FACE AND HEAD

The face and head have an extremely rich arterial supply (**Figures 49 and 50**). The anastomosis between the two sides is so good that if a facial artery or one of its branches is cut, both ends of the cut vessel show pulsatile bleeding, instead of only the cardiac end as elsewhere.

The **facial artery** is the main superficial artery to the face. It leaves the external carotid artery just behind the angle of the mandible, immediately after the lingual (which runs deep to the mandible to supply the tongue, where its pulsations can often be seen or felt on the underside of the tip). The facial artery then loops up and down behind the submandibular gland, grooving it posteriorly and supplying it. It then runs over the surface of the gland and then over the mandible at the anterior border of the masseter muscle. If the jaw is clenched, the anterior border of the muscle becomes palpable, with the facial artery pulsating over the bone (**Figure 51**). The facial vein accompanies the artery, together with the mandibular branch of the facial nerve and lymphatics. In facial inflammation, a lymph node may become palpable here.

From the mandible, the artery follows an irregular course across the face to the inner canthus of the eye, giving branches as it goes, to the upper and lower lips and nose, and linking with the deeper transverse facial artery. The branches to the lips are large, and the pulsations of the anastomosed arteries may be felt by holding the lip between finger and thumb.

The **superficial temporal artery** is the other major artery whose pulsations can easily be felt in the face. It is the continuation of the external carotid artery after its last branch, the maxillary, has left it in the substance of the parotid gland, to run forwards deep to the neck of the mandible. The superficial temporal artery runs anterior to the ear, over the zygomatic arch, where it is palpable (**Figure 52**). The artery passes over the temporal fascia to divide into frontal and parietal branches, the former supplying the forehead and the latter supplying the parietal scalp, each anastomosing with branches of the opposite side.

The **supraorbital and supratrochlear arteries** are branches of the ophthalmic, which leave the orbit, pierce the frontalis muscle and run up onto the forehead. Pulsations of the supraorbital artery can usually be felt about 2.5 cm from the midline (see *supraorbital nerve*, page 20).

The **occipital artery** supplies the posterior part of the scalp. It appears from beneath sternomastoid and runs onto the scalp, between that muscle and trapezius. It can readily be felt as it crosses the superior nuchal line, four fingers' breadth behind the ear.

The rich vascularity of the face allows remarkable liberty in movement of tissue by **flaps** for local surgical repair. A **superficial temporal artery flap** allows the whole forehead to be transposed on the frontal branch for repair of the cheek or chin, whereas, particularly in a bald person, the anterior scalp can likewise be moved on the parietal branch (**Figure 50**), the defect in the scalp being repaired by a split skin graft. Very narrowly based flaps on the **supratrochlear or supraorbital vessels** allow quite long **forehead flaps** to be turned down to repair the nose

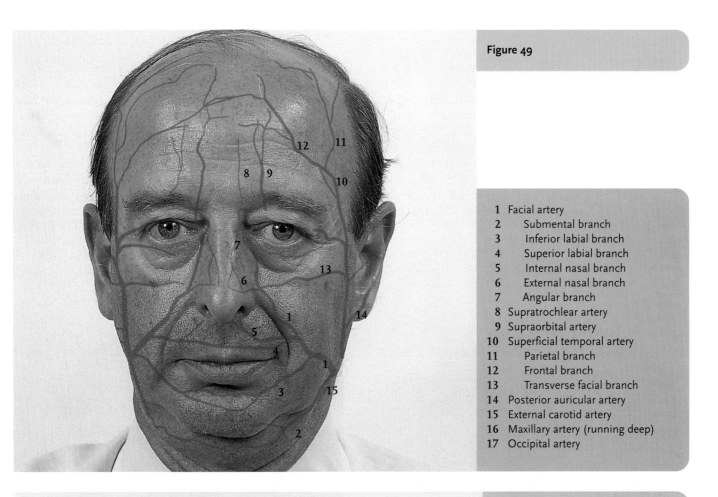

Figure 49

1 Facial artery
2   Submental branch
3   Inferior labial branch
4   Superior labial branch
5   Internal nasal branch
6   External nasal branch
7   Angular branch
8 Supratrochlear artery
9 Supraorbital artery
10 Superficial temporal artery
11   Parietal branch
12   Frontal branch
13   Transverse facial branch
14 Posterior auricular artery
15 External carotid artery
16 Maxillary artery (running deep)
17 Occipital artery

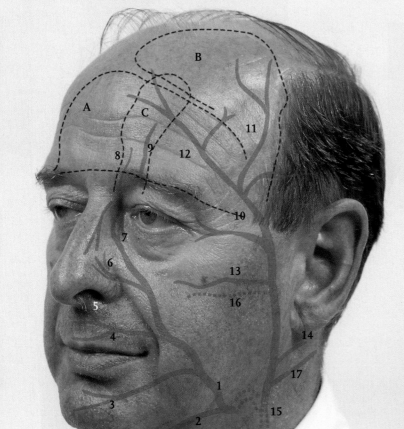

Figure 50

A Whole forehead flap including
  frontal branch of superficial
  temporal artery
B Anterior scalp flap on parietal
  branch of superficial temporal artery
C Forehead flap on supratrochlear
  bland supraorbital vessels
(Numbered as Figure 49)

or the adjoining area. So rich is the supply in the face that quite narrowly based flaps can be taken, even without great regard for vessels, in a way that is impossible elsewhere in the body.

The **middle meningeal artery** is an important artery that may rupture intracranially in head injury. It enters the skull through the foramen spinosum, which is level with the middle of the upper border of the zygomatic arch. It then follows a course laterally within the skull for a variable distance before dividing into frontal and parietal branches. From the lateral side, this will only be a few millimetres above the point of entry into the skull. The frontal or anterior channel then runs almost vertically, while the parietal (posterior) branch runs backwards and slightly upwards.

THE SALIVARY GLANDS

The major paired salivary glands are the parotid (mainly serous), the submandibular (mixed serous and mucous) and the sublingual (mainly mucous). Many small glands are scattered around the mouth in the palate, cheeks, lips, the posterior part of the dorsum, and the periphery and underside of the tongue.

The **parotid** has its major part in the space between the anterior aspect of the mastoid process and sternomastoid muscle, and the ramus of the mandible. Superiorly, it runs up to the external auditory meatus and down almost to the angle of the mandible. Deeply, it is limited by the styloid process

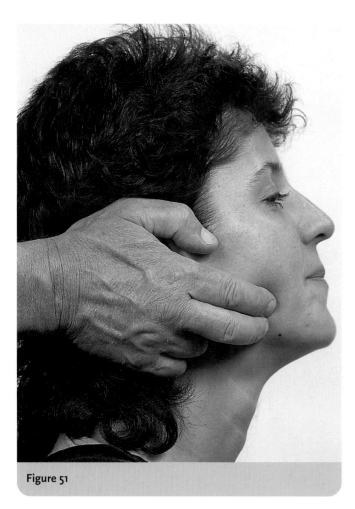

Figure 51

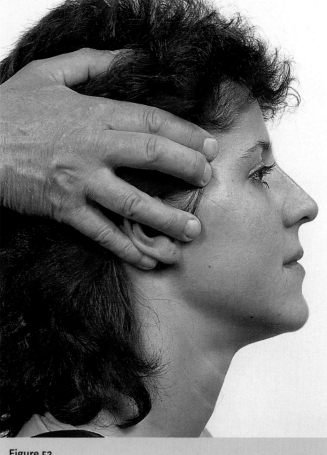

Figure 52

and the stylomandibular ligament, but it can come close to the pharyngeal wall. The superficial portion goes forwards over the surface of the masseter onto the cheek (**Figure 53**). Because of its dense capsule, which is continuous with the masseteric fascia, it is not easy to feel in the normal state, though the lower border may be identified. Therefore, any readily palpable gland is probably pathological. Occasionally, lymph glands may become palpable over the surface of the gland and at the anterior border of the masseter.

The **parotid duct** runs forwards, level with the upper part of the ear lobe, and opens inside the cheek, level with the second upper molar tooth. The opening is usually visible, where a cannula can be passed if needed.

The **submandibular gland** lies superficially beneath the mandible, in a hollow in front of the angle and in the space between it and mylohyoid muscle, where the outlines of the gland may be felt by careful examination (**Figure 53**). The duct runs forwards, deep to mylohyoid, and opens at the **sublingual papilla**, with the several openings of the sublingual gland (**Figure 54**). Superficial to the gland, submandibular lymph nodes may be felt if these become swollen.

The **sublingual gland** lies superficially in the floor of the mouth, deep to the mucosa of the sublingual fold, to the side of the frenulum (**Figure 54**).

1 Parotid gland
2 Parotid duct
3 Submandibular gland
4 Angle of the mandible
5 Hyoid bone
6 Digastric muscle
7 Thyroid cartilage
8 Sternomastoid muscle

1 Underside of tongue
2 Plica fimbriata
3 Frenulum linguae
4 Lingual vein overlying lingual gland
5 Sublingual papillae
6 Sublingual fold over sublingual gland

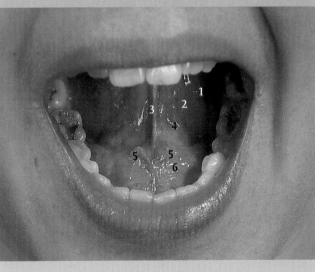

Figure 54

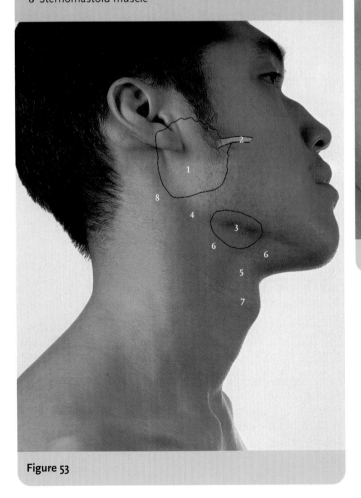

Figure 53

Chapter 3

The neck

The neck is the highly mobile upper end of the trunk, which generates the relatively free mobility of the head (**Figure 55A–C**). Consequently, the muscles and joints of the neck have the fine neural control that is needed to ensure the delicate balance and movement control of the head on the trunk. Unfortunately, the mobility also permits bad posture, and—usually because of this—osteoarthrosis of the cervical vertebrae is common and often extensive, with neurological damage.

Sternomastoid muscle runs downwards and forwards, from the mastoid process and superior nuchal line of the skull to the manubrium sterni and the clavicle. An anteromedial portion forms a round tendon running to the manubrium, which stands out when the muscle contracts. The lateral component remains as muscle, running to the medial third of the

clavicle, and is less obvious on contraction (**Figure 56**). Contraction of a single muscle turns the head to the opposite side and facing upwards. Resistance from a hand can enhance the effect. Contraction of both muscles pulls the back of the head downwards and the neck forwards (cranes the head).

When both sternomastoid muscles are contracted, the suprasternal hollow is emphasised (**Figure 56**).

Contraction of a single sternomastoid to turn the head is usually accompanied by contraction of the upper fibres of trapezius, which enhances the intervening **supraclavicular fossa**, the base of the posterior triangle of the neck (**Figure 57**). The **posterior triangle** has its apex at the junction of these muscles at the superior nuchal line, where the occipital artery can be felt pulsating, having emerged from beneath sternomastoid to run up onto the scalp. **Splenius capitis** and **levator**

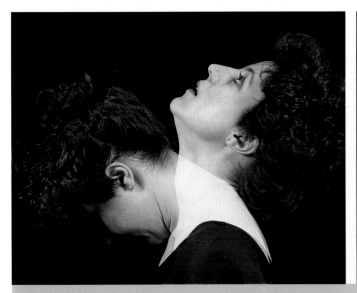

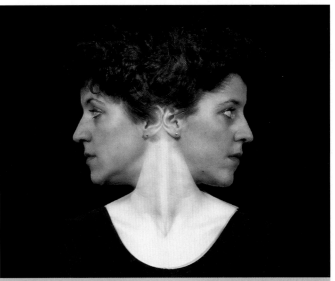

Figure 55A and B Flexion and extension are remarkably free, allowing flexion to bring the chin onto the chest and a considerable range of extension limited by the neural arches and muscle control.

Rotation occurs throughout the neck, with some 60–80° in each direction. About half this rotation occurs between the axis and atlas vertebrae, with the other half in the remainder of the neck.

scapulae form the floor of the upper part of the triangle, though they lie mainly beneath trapezius. **Scalenus medius** forms the greater part, running from the posterior tubercles of all the cervical transverse processes (usually) down to the first rib. More anteriorly, the **scalenus anterior** completes the floor, with the **phrenic nerve** running down over its surface.

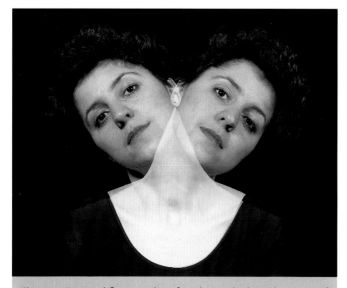

Figure 55C Lateral flexion is less free due to the lateral masses of the vertebrae, but if a little rotation is allowed, the range is very much increased. Note that a small amount of rotation has occurred in this case to allow the range achieved.

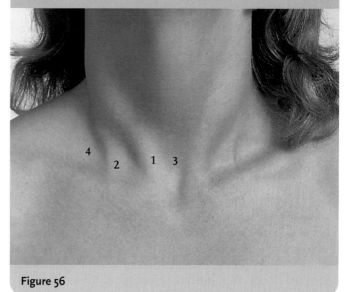

1 Sternal head of sternomastoid
2 Clavicular head of sternomastoid
3 Suprasternal notch
4 Supraclavicular fossa

Figure 56

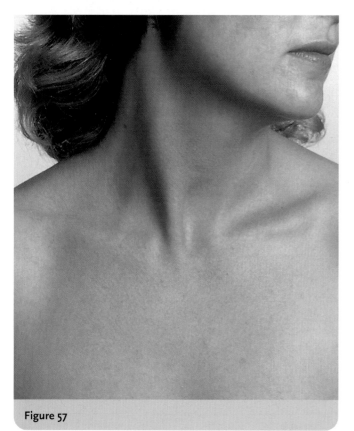

Figure 57

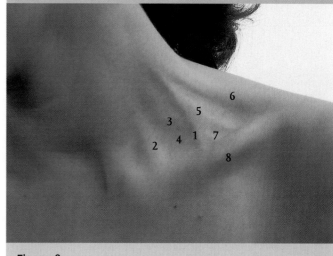

1 External jugular vein
2 Posterior border of sternomastoid
3 Omohyoid muscle
4 Scalenus anterior (crossed by phrenic nerve)
5 Scalenus medius
6 Anterior border of trapezius
7 Brachial plexus
8 Clavicle

Figure 58

The roots and trunks of the **brachial plexus** run down from between the two scalene muscles to pass deep to the clavicle and may raise a ridge when the head is leant to the opposite side. The external jugular vein runs down the triangle, where it may be readily visible (often over the brachial plexus), and passes deep to the clavicle, joining the subclavian or the internal jugular vein (**Figure 58**).

The **omohyoid muscle and tendon** run obliquely downwards and posteriorly across the triangle, from beneath the sternomastoid, about level with the cricoid cartilage, to its insertion by the suprascapular notch. They may produce a ridge if the shoulders are raised.

If the finger is pressed down behind the middle of the clavicle, the **subclavian artery** should be felt pulsating against the first rib, or even against the transverse process of C6 in those cases where it makes a high loop. Pressure behind the clavicle can also compress the trunks of the brachial plexus, giving the recipient that strange feeling of nerve compression.

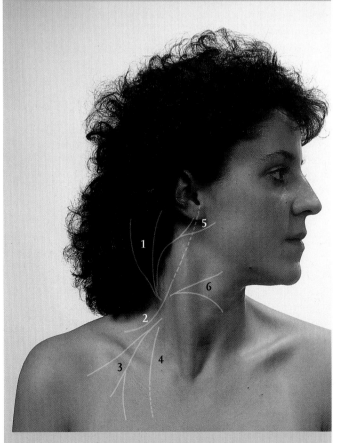

1 Greater and lesser occipital
2 Accessory
3 Supraclavicular
4 Phrenic
5 Greater auricular
6 Transverse cervical

Figure 59 Cervical nerves.

The **accessory nerve** runs across the triangle, from midway down the posterior border of sternomastoid to the anterior border of trapezius, about 5 cm above the clavicle. The various C4 **supraclavicular nerves** emerge from behind the sternomastoid at about the same point, and runs down over the clavicle, where they can sometimes be felt by rolling the finger on the bone (**Figure 59**).

Supraclavicular lymph nodes lie in the supraclavicular fossa and, if swollen, may become apparent.

CERVICAL NERVES

These give—as do most spinal nerves—both anterior and posterior primary rami, the latter supplying the vertebral muscles and the overlying skin. C1 is entirely muscular. C2 gives wider sensory supply, forming the **greater occipital nerve**, which pierces trapezius to supply the back of the head. It can usually be palpated as it crosses the superior nuchal line, close to the attachment of trapezius, about midway between the mastoid process and the midline. It may be involved in neural pressure at this site due to muscle tension, giving headache, which is often migrainous in character.

The anterior primary rami of the **upper four cervical nerves** form a plexus, supplying cervical musculature and skin of the neck and (C4) the shoulders. The **phrenic nerve** arises mainly from C4, with small contributions from C3 and larger ones from C5, giving all the motor and most (60%) of the sensory supply to the diaphragm.

C2 arises above the transverse process of the axis, and C3 and C4 above their respective vertebrae. The major branches appear behind sternomastoid (**Figure 59**). The **supraclavicular nerves** leave at about the middle of the muscle, as does the **accessory nerve**. A little higher, the **greater auricular** (C2–C3) turns upwards and anteriorly over the muscle, towards the angle of the mandible, supplying the skin overlying the angle and the parotid gland, the lower $^2/_3$ or so of the back of the ear plus the lobular region and a little above, anteriorly.

Cervical nerve block depends upon the localisation of the transverse processes of the cervical vertebrae (**Figure 60**), which are relatively superficial. That of C2 is about 1 cm below the mastoid process. That of C4 is at about the middle and just behind the posterior border of sternomastoid, where the external jugular vein usually runs over its surface. C6 can be felt above the middle of the clavicle, the so-called carotid tubercle.

Anaesthesia of the cervical roots is also likely to block the cervical sympathetic chain, producing lid lag on that side.

The **phrenic** nerve runs down over the surface of scalenus anterior, behind the lower part of sternomastoid. If the clavicular head of sternomastoid is pulled forwards, and the area towards the anterior tubercle of C6 infiltrated, the nerve should be effectively anaesthetised (**Figure 61**). Conversely, the phrenic nerve can be stimulated electrically to induce diaphragmatic respiratory movement by applying the electrodes at the same site as for injection.

The roots and trunks of the **brachial plexus** lie in the posterior triangle of the neck, the divisions behind the clavicle and the cords in the axilla. The upper and middle trunks are readily accessible in the triangle, but the lower trunk lies close to the first rib, behind the clavicle. If a line is drawn from the middle of the posterior border of the sternomastoid to the middle of the clavicle, this should overlie the trunks and roots, beginning with C5 (plus usually some of C4) down to T1 beneath the clavicle. If the head is held to the opposite side, a ridge raised by the trunks should be palpable and even visible (**Figure 58**).

Local **nerve block of the brachial plexus** can be done at several sites. A supraclavicular approach is excellent, but there is often anxiety over the danger of pneumothorax caused by the needle perforating the suprapleural membrane (Sibson's fascia) and the pleura if the syringe is carelessly disconnected from the needle. At the midpoint of the clavicle, the external jugular vein passes beneath it and pulsations of the subclavian artery may be felt (**Figure 62**). The plexus should run immediately behind the pulse, but it is usual to make the injection 1–2 cm above the clavicle, pointing downwards and backwards. It is important to be sure, as always, that the needle is not in a vessel or, here, in the lung. To avoid the risk of penetrating the lung, a somewhat higher interscalene injection is often preferred. It is important that the injection is within the

fascial sheath of the plexus, to allow the anaesthetic to track down to lower levels.

An axillary approach to the plexus is also possible, but the disadvantage here is the spread-out nature of the cords around the artery, large veins also being a problem.

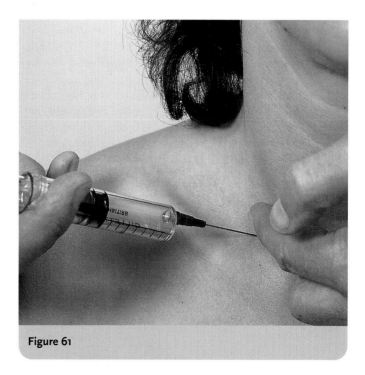

Figure 61

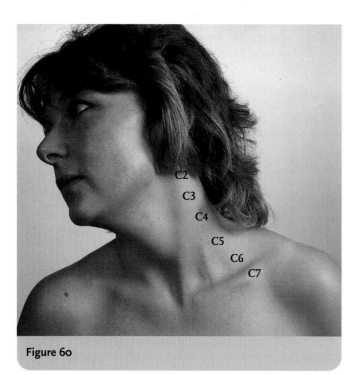

Figure 60

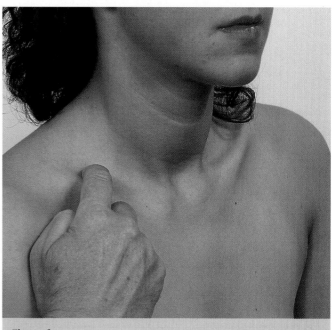

Figure 62

THE GREAT ARTERIES OF THE NECK

The neck is an important transit zone for vessels linking the heart with the brain, as well as for local head and neck supply.

The **vertebral vessels**, including the rich vertebral venous plexus, supply much of the brain, as well as the cervical spinal cord and vertebral region. The vertebral artery, from the first part of the subclavian, usually enters the foramen transversarium of the sixth cervical vertebra, the transverse process of which can be felt a little above the middle of the clavicle.

The **common carotid arteries** run upwards. The right side is formed behind the sternoclavicular joint, by division of the brachiocephalic into it and the subclavian artery. On the left side, the common carotid leaves the arch of the aorta behind the left side of the manubrium sterni and then runs upwards behind the sternoclavicular joint. The arteries then follow a more or less straight course upwards, towards the ear, where the internal carotid branch enters the skull, about 1 cm deep to and a little behind the head of the mandible (or deep to the intertragic notch of the ear) (**Figure 63**).

The common carotid artery normally divides behind the superior cornu of the thyroid cartilage, into internal and external branches (**Figure 63**). The **external carotid artery** runs at first anteromedial to the **internal carotid** and later more lateral, ending within the parotid gland, behind and deep to the neck of the mandible. Here it divides into its terminal branches; the superficial temporal continues in line over the zygomatic arch (see page 24), while the maxillary artery runs directly forwards, deep to the neck of the mandible.

The first branch of the external carotid artery, the **superior thyroid artery**, leaves to run to the upper pole of the thyroid gland (in consort with the superior laryngeal nerve), either after or just before the division. The **ascending pharyngeal** leaves the medial aspect shortly thereafter. The **lingual artery** leaves the anterior aspect at about the level of the greater cornu of the hyoid bone, followed almost immediately by the **facial artery**, usually tucked under cover of the angle of the mandible before looping onto the face (see pages 24 and 25). Just above the greater cornu of the hyoid bone, the **occipital** artery runs backwards under cover of the sternomastoid muscle, to appear on the scalp just medial to its attachment. As the occipital artery leaves, the **hypoglossal nerve** appears from between the arteries and the internal jugular vein, loops round the origin of the occipital artery and then runs forwards over the external carotid, under cover of the posterior belly of the digastric

1 Common carotid
2 External carotid
3 Internal carotid
4 Superior thyroid
5 Lingual
6 Facial
7 Maxillary
8 Superficial temporal
9 Occipital
10 Posterior auricular

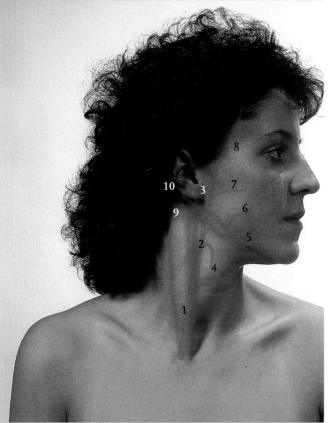

Figure 63 Common carotid artery and its branches.

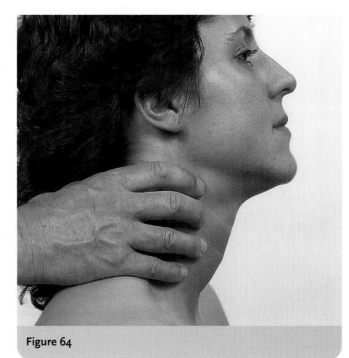

Figure 64

muscle. The **posterior auricular artery** runs backwards from the external carotid shortly after the occipital (or may leave with it as a common stem), entering the parotid gland to reach its final destination.

The **carotid sinus and body** are both found at the division of the common carotid artery, and so are close to and just behind the superior cornu of the thyroid cartilage.

The carotid arteries can be felt pulsating in the neck by pressing in front of the sternomastoid muscle, towards the transverse processes of the cervical vertebrae (**Figure 64**, see previous page).

THE GREAT VEINS OF THE NECK

The major venous channel from the brain, other than the important vertebral venous plexus and vein, is the **internal jugular vein (Figure 65A)**. It leaves the skull as a continuation

of the **sigmoid sinus** through the jugular foramen, just lateral to and a few millimetres behind the internal carotid artery, deep to the intertragic notch of the ear. It runs down with the internal and then the common carotid arteries (and the vagus nerve), passing deep to sternomastoid in the lower half of the neck, where it lies lateral to the artery. In the root of the neck, it crosses in front of the subclavian artery and joins the subclavian vein behind the sternoclavicular joint, to become the **brachiocephalic vein**. That on the left side crosses close behind the upper half of the manubrium sterni, joining the right, which then runs down as the **superior vena cava**.

The internal jugular vein receives the **facial vein** and a branch from the **retromandibular vein** a little below the angle of the mandible, usually together with the **superior thyroid**, **lingual** and **pharyngeal veins**. A little lower, about level with the cricoid, a **middle thyroid vein** may join it. Although not always present (about 50% of cases), it is of great importance

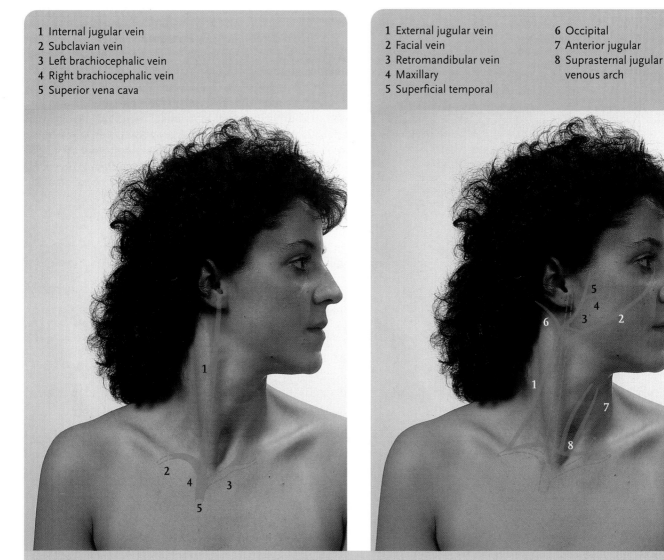

1 Internal jugular vein
2 Subclavian vein
3 Left brachiocephalic vein
4 Right brachiocephalic vein
5 Superior vena cava

1 External jugular vein   6 Occipital
2 Facial vein   7 Anterior jugular
3 Retromandibular vein   8 Suprasternal jugular
4 Maxillary   venous arch
5 Superficial temporal

Figure 65A and B

surgically. It is a short vein running straight over the common carotid artery to the internal jugular vein, from which it may easily be torn, while mobilising the tissues, in thyroidectomy.

The **external jugular vein** (**Figure 65B**) begins in the parotid gland, most commonly by union of the superficial temporal and maxillary veins, together with the posterior auricular and a link branch with the facial. It runs down from behind the angle of the mandible, over the surface of sternomastoid muscle, sinks behind the middle of the clavicle, and joins the subclavian vein or, in about 30% of cases, the internal jugular vein. It is usually visible in its course down the neck (**Figure 58**), particularly when engorged.

Anterior jugular veins run down from the submental region, following a variable course to the lower neck, where in the suprasternal notch they are usually joined by a **jugular venous arch**. In view of the jugular venous arch, the inferior thyroid veins (draining into the left brachiocephalic) and the deeper position of the trachea, this is an unsuitable place for an **emergency tracheostomy**, although excellent for an elective procedure. The emergency approach should be above, where the larynx and trachea are superficial and have no overlying structures in the midline. The choice rests with cutting between the thyroid and cricoid cartilages, i.e. a **laryngostomy** (the disadvantage being risk of scars of the cords), or through the upper rings of the trachea (**high tracheostomy**), either dividing or pulling down the isthmus of the thyroid gland.

CENTRAL VENOUS CATHETERISATION

Knowledge of the sites of ready approach to the veins is important. Although the veins at the antecubital fossa are useful, there may be difficulty in threading the catheter through the veins to the heart. An approach through the internal jugular or subclavian vein may be needed, the right side giving easier passage to the heart. Accurate positioning of the needle is vital to prevent unnecessary damage to these important veins.

The **internal jugular vein** runs deep to the sternomastoid muscle in the lower part of the neck (**Figure 66**), and so it can be approached about midway down the anterior border of the muscle, just lateral to the carotid pulse (**1**). Although the vein is behind sternomastoid, the muscle divides into sternal and clavicular attachments, leaving a gap through which the needle can be passed in a downwards and medial direction (**2**). This position is better in a conscious patient.

Alternatively, the **subclavian vein** may be approached as it runs over the first rib and behind the medial third of the clavicle, either from above the clavicle (**3**) or below (**4**). The available position is at the junction of the intermediate and medial thirds of the clavicle. From above, this will be at the lateral border of sternomastoid, and the needle passes downwards and medially; from below, it is passed upwards and omedially. In either case it is important to remember that the vein runs close behind the clavicle.

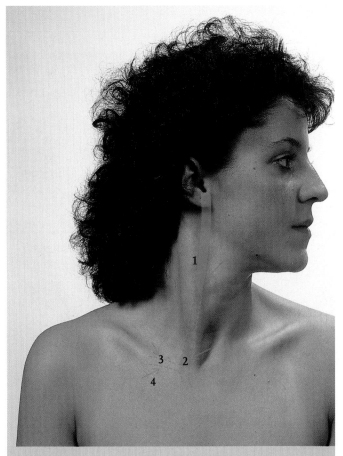

Figure 66 The internal jugular vein runs deep to the lower part of the sternomastoid muscle in the lower part of the neck and so it can be approached about midway down the anterior border of the muscle just lateral to the carotid pulse (**1**). Although the vein is behind sternomastoid, this muscle divides into sternal and clavicular attachments, leaving a gap through which the needle can be passed in a downwards and medial direction (**2**). This position is better in a conscious patient. Alternatively, the subclavian vein may be approached as it runs over the first rib, behind the medial third of the clavicle (**3**) or below (**4**).

LYMPHATICS OF THE HEAD AND NECK

The lymph glands are not normally palpable, but it is important to know where to examine in case of swelling, from either infection or malignancy (**Figure 67**).

    Superficial glands are found around the face and head: on the cheek at the anterior border of masseter, on the parotid, and over the mastoid and occipital regions of the head. At a slightly lower level, **submental glands** drain the tip of the tongue, the lower lip and mouth, while the **submandibular glands** receive from the submental and from the tongue, mouth, cheek, upper lip and nasal cavity. More posterior lymphatics drain into glands along the **external jugular vein** which, in turn, drain into the deep cervical nodes, as do lymphatics from the pharyngeal and tracheal regions.

The **deep cervical nodes** lie along the internal jugular vein and form the main collecting system for the head and neck. They are usually described as **superior and inferior deep cervical groups**. The former group includes the **jugulodigastric or tonsillar node**; the latter, the **jugulo-omohyoid node**. The majority of the nodes lie deep to the sternomastoid muscle, which has lymphatics running in its fascial sheath. (Hence, in functional block dissection of the neck for malignancy, the fascia is stripped, leaving the muscle and accessory nerve intact.) The anterior of the superior nodes, including the jugulodigastric, can be felt anterior to the upper part of sternomastoid; the posterior of the lower group may be felt along the posterior border of the muscle, i.e. in the posterior triangle, where **supraclavicular nodes** may also be felt, in the hollow above the clavicle.

1 Occipital
2 Superficial cervical
3 Supraclavicular
4 Parotid
5 Submandibular
6 Submental
7 Superior deep cervical
8 Anterior cervical and midline nodes
9 Inferior deep cervical

1 Mandible
2 Submandibular gland
3 Hyoid bone
4 Posterior belly of digastric
5 Anterior belly of digastric
6 Anterior border of masseter
7 Thyroid cartilage
8 Superior cornu of thyroid cartilage

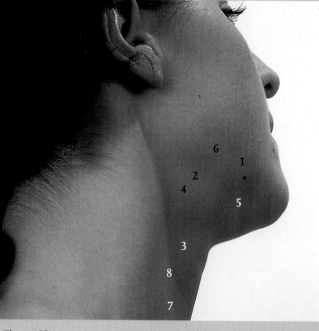

Figure 68

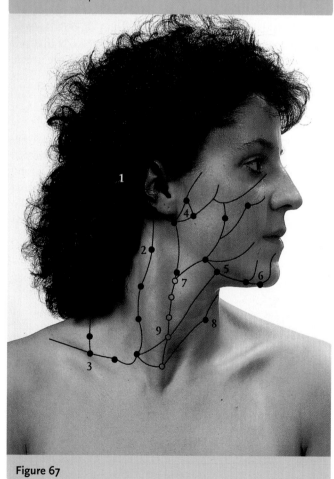

Figure 67

THE SUBMANDIBULAR REGION

In a young person, when the skin is put on stretch, it is often possible to identify a number of structures, and these can be used as indicators for the whereabouts of others (**Figure 68**). However, this is a region where subcutaneous fat may be laid down and where the skin sags with ageing, both of which may effectively camouflage the structures.

THE LARYNX

The laryngeal prominence is often visible in the neck as 'Adam's apple'. This, as the name implies, is most obvious in adult males due to its larger size (**Figure 69**). The visible component is the **thyroid cartilage**, with its upper border and the vertically running angle between the two laminae. The **vocal cords or ligaments** are attached to the back of the thyroid cartilage and run backwards to the **arytenoid cartilages**, mounted on the posterior lamina of the **cricoid**.

The male larynx grows at puberty, so that the cords which are some 12.5–17 mm in a prepubertal child or a woman are some 17–23 mm in men. The thyroid cartilage thus projects farther forwards and its angle becomes sharper, from 120° in a child or woman to 90° in a man.

If the head is fully extended (**Figure 70**), the upper part of the thyroid cartilage is midway between chin and sternum, but in a natural position it lies closely under the chin. In an adult the cricoid cartilage is level with the sixth cervical vertebra, and the hyoid bone level with C3–C4. In a newborn baby the larynx is much higher, with the epiglottis level with the soft palate, but it sinks as the face and neck grow. The high position of the infant larynx, together with large glandular swellings in the aryepiglottic folds (which effectively raise and seal the larynx posteriorly), permits the milk to pass around the larynx until effective cough reflex and neuromuscular control are developed.

Palpation of the larynx should be carried out very gently. Gentle palpation not only increases tactile sensibility in the operator, but also avoids pressure on the larynx, particularly in the cricoid region, which can produce an unpleasant sensation for the patient.

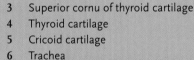

1	Hyoid bone
2	Thyro-hyoid membrane
3	Superior cornu of thyroid cartilage
4	Thyroid cartilage
5	Cricoid cartilage
6	Trachea

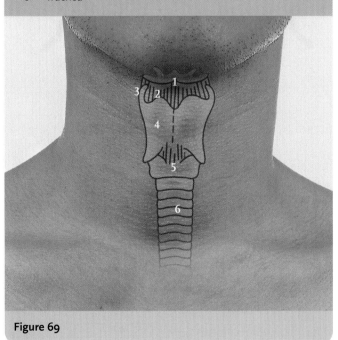

Figure 69

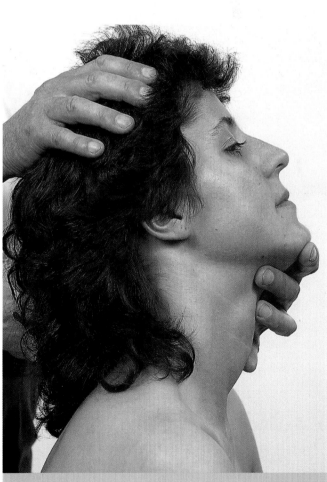

Figure 70 The examiner's index finger rests on the chin, the middle finger to the side of the hyoid bone, the ring finger on the upper part of the thyroid cartilage, and the little finger on the cricoid.

The **hyoid bone** is a base for muscle attachments and, most importantly, is there to keep open the lateral food channels (i.e. the pyriform fossae) around the larynx. Because of its muscle attachments, both above and below, it is not easy to palpate anteriorly; however, if the finger is moved more to the side, it becomes easier (**Figure 70**). The two greater cornua may be taken gently between the finger and thumb, tucked closely under the mandible. If the finger is carried down from the hyoid, it comes to rest on the projecting shelf of the thyroid cartilage. If carried down the vertical angle of the thyroid cartilage, it will come to a shallow depression before meeting another slight prominence, the anterior arch of the cricoid.

THE THYROID GLAND

The strap muscles of the neck run down on either side of the midline from the hyoid to the sternum and cover the lobes of the thyroid gland. However, with gentle palpation it is often possible to feel the slight thickening produced by the isthmus of the gland crossing the second and third tracheal rings, just below the cricoid swelling. The lower aspect of each isthmus can often be seen bulging slightly, forming an upper feature of the suprasternal notch. This is more likely in an older male, owing to the more prominent larynx and thinner skin (**Figure 72**).

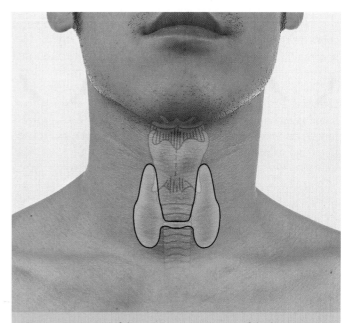

Figure 72 Because of the greater prominence of the larynx in a male, it is sometimes possible to see the outlines of the thyroid gland to some extent even when normal.

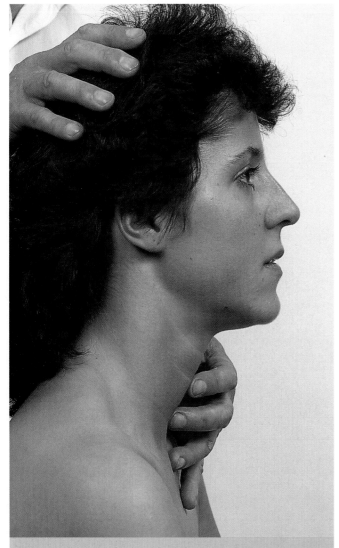

Figure 71 The index finger rests in the hollow between the thyroid and cricoid cartilages, the middle finger on the isthmus of the thyroid gland, the ring finger on the suprasternal notch, and the little finger over the manubriosternal joint (sternal angle of Louis).

Chapter 4
Shoulder girdle and arm

The shoulder girdle is essentially the scapula with an anterior limb, the clavicle, which has the only true joint with the trunk. Its design is for finely controlled mobility and a base for the further activity of the arms.

The **sternoclavicular joint** is essentially non-loadbearing, being divided into two parts by a fibrocartilaginous disc. The axis of movement is some 2–3 mm along the bone, around the attachment of the costoclavicular ligament, with control from the subclavius muscle. The medial end of the clavicle therefore shows considerable mobility relative to the manubrium sterni in movement of the girdle.

The **clavicle** curves around the upper chest wall, overlying the **first rib (making it impalpable)**. The lateral part shows a reverse curve, producing the hollow to the shoulder. The lateral end joins the **acromion**, a curved continuation of the **spine of the scapula**.

The **acromioclavicular joint** has minimal movement; the clavicle and scapula moving virtually in unison on the trunk, around the costoclavicular axis. The bony continuum of the clavicle and the acromion and spine of the scapula are normally palpable and often visible (**Figure 73**). The inferior angle of the scapula is usually obvious, particularly if the shoulder is moved (**Figure 75**).

The **coracoid process** of the scapula may be felt below the lateral aspect of the clavicle, through the anterior fibres of deltoid muscle. Medial to deltoid is a small gap between it and

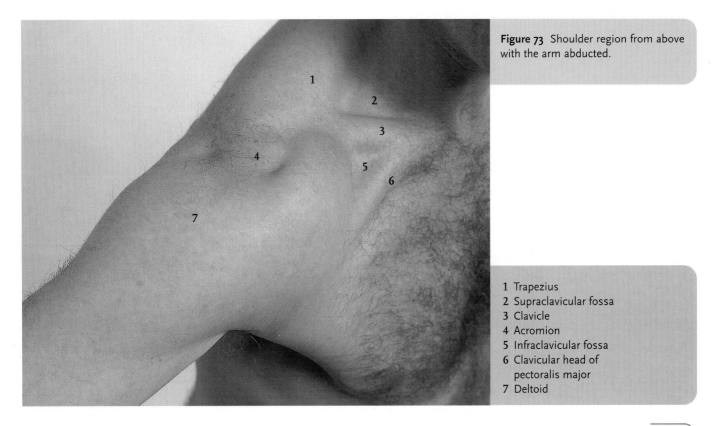

Figure 73 Shoulder region from above with the arm abducted.

1 Trapezius
2 Supraclavicular fossa
3 Clavicle
4 Acromion
5 Infraclavicular fossa
6 Clavicular head of pectoralis major
7 Deltoid

the clavicular head of pectoralis major, the **infraclavicular fossa**, continuous below with the **deltopectoral groove**, which runs across the front of the shoulder, containing the cephalic vein (**Figure 74**).

The **shoulder joint** lies beneath the deltoid muscle, but palpation a little below the acromion may allow the two humeral tuberosities to be felt, particularly if the arm is rotated, to help identify the contour changes. In the the anatomical position (i.e. with the palm of the hand facing forwards), the greater tuberosity lies laterally and the lesser lies anteriorly; however, in the normal functional position, the greater tuberosity lies anteriorly, with the lesser medial.

The large rounded humeral head fits to a shallow glenoid fossa, so that this joint, like the shoulder girdle, depends upon its controlling muscles for stability. The fine neuromuscular control so needed probably explains why relatively minor injuries around the joint often produce severe problem, e.g. frozen shoulder.

Examination of movements at the shoulder must identify those between girdle and trunk, and those at the shoulder joint. Some movements are a combination of both, and with some common muscles, their clinical separation often presents problems.

At the **shoulder girdle**, elevation and depression indicate movements of the scapula without rotation. Protraction carries the scapula around the chest wall, bringing the shoulder forwards, whereas retraction pulls the scapula towards the spine ('braces the shoulder'). Upward and downward rotation of the scapula indicates the direction of movement of the glenoid fossa; normally components of abduction and adduction of the arm, they can be produced separately (**Figure 75**).

Movements at the shoulder joint are registered relative to the normal position of the scapula, i.e. with the glenoid facing slightly forwards, so that abduction and adduction are a little anterior to the plane of the trunk. Abduction of the arm is a combined movement at both systems; a little over 90°

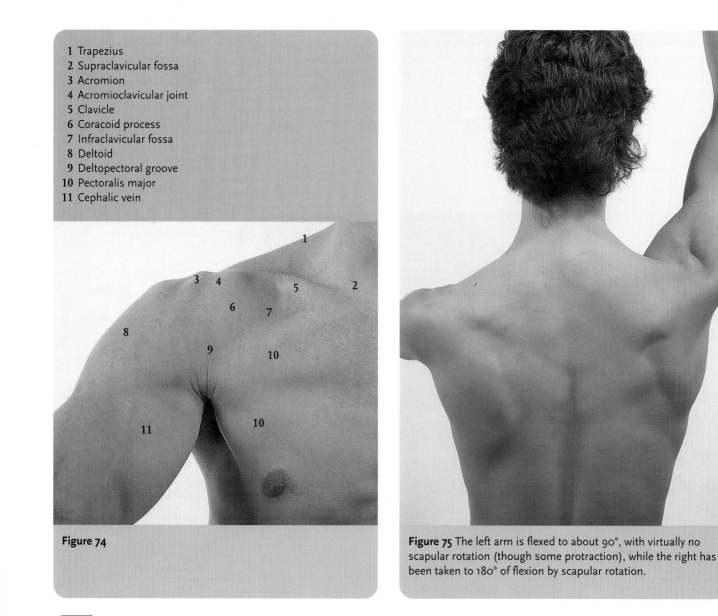

1 Trapezius
2 Supraclavicular fossa
3 Acromion
4 Acromioclavicular joint
5 Clavicle
6 Coracoid process
7 Infraclavicular fossa
8 Deltoid
9 Deltopectoral groove
10 Pectoralis major
11 Cephalic vein

Figure 74

Figure 75 The left arm is flexed to about 90°, with virtually no scapular rotation (though some protraction), while the right has been taken to 180° of flexion by scapular rotation.

being possible at the shoulder joint, the remainder coming from rotation of the scapula. Although there is individual variation, the shoulder joint contributes the greater amount initially, as the arm moves from the side (**Figure 75**).

Flexion and extension are at right angles to the plane of the scapula. Flexion is mainly at the shoulder joint for some 90°, but added range comes from rotation of the scapula (**Figure 75**).

Medial and lateral rotation at the shoulder joint are also important and powerful movements (see pages 49–51).

MUSCLES CONTROLLING THE SHOULDER GIRDLE

Two muscles run to the clavicle from the head and neck. **Sternomastoid** joins its medial third (page 29). **Trapezius** is attached to its lateral third, to the acromion and to the spine of the scapula. It is a large triangular muscle covering the neck and shoulder regions, the muscles on the two sides together forming a trapezium. It has a long attachment to the superior nuchal line of the occiput (medial to sternomastoid), the ligamentum nuchae in the neck, and the spines and supraspinous ligaments of the seventh cervical and all the thoracic vertebrae. The cranial fibres run to the clavicle, with the lower fibres being attached progressively to the acromion and along the spine of the scapula to its medial end. The cranial fibres can either extend the head on the neck, turning it to the opposite side or, if the head is fixed, raise the point of the shoulder; the intermediate fibres will brace the shoulders (retract the scapula), while the lowest will pull the medial aspect of the scapula downwards. Each part can act separately with other muscles of a similar function, or the whole muscle will rotate the scapula upwards, as in abduction of the arm (**Figure 76**). It can give useful movement of the arm even after arthrodesis (fixation) of the shoulder joint.

Trapezius is vital for postural support of the shoulder girdle. It receives motor innervation from the spinal accessory nerve, with sensory fibres from C3–C4. Loss of the spinal accessory nerve, as after a classical lymph gland block dissection of the neck (which removes sternomastoid), usually leads to severe dropping of the shoulder, with the scapula rotating downwards under the weight of the arm. (This is not always so, probably due to some motor fibres carried in the mainly sensory C3–C4 supply.) **Levator scapulae**, running from the cervical vertebrae, under trapezius, to the upper border of the scapula, is the other **elevator** of the scapula;

1 Upper fibres of trapezius (contracting firmly on right)
2 Middle fibres of trapezius (contracting firmly on right)
3 Lower fibres of trapezius (contracting firmly on right)
4 Rhomboideus major
5 Spine of scapula
6 Supraspinatus bulging under trapezius
7 Deltoid
8 Infraspinatus
9 Teres minor
10 Teres major
11 Latissimus dorsi

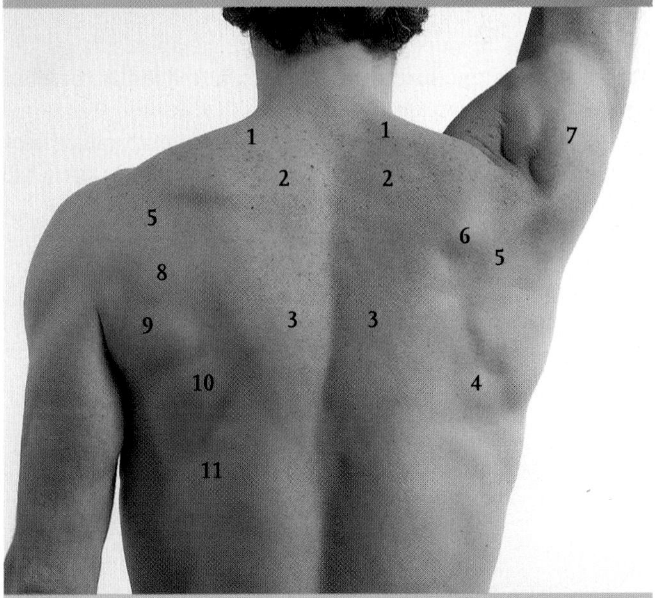

Figure 76 The right arm has been abducted through 180° with the left in normal resting position. The right scapula has been rotated through 70–75° by trapezius, the remaining movement occurring at the shoulder joint. Activity is obvious in deltoid, the main abductor at the shoulder joint, but that in supraspinatus is masked by the overlying trapezius.

it gives only secondary and more medial support (**Figure 77**). **Depression** of the scapula is brought about by the lower fibres of trapezius, together with latissimus dorsi acting on the humerus. **Retraction** of the scapula (bracing the shoulders) is controlled by the intermediate fibres of trapezius, together with the **rhomboids** lying beneath (**Figure 78**). Loss of the nerve supply to the rhomboids (C5) allows the scapula to fall away from the chest because of the pull of the arm muscles arising from the scapula, giving particular prominence to the angle of the scapula.

    Protraction of the scapula is produced by **serratus anterior**. It arises by digitations from the upper eight ribs (**Figure 79**) and runs back around the chest wall, beneath the scapula, to be attached to its medial border. Posturally, with the rhomboids, it holds the scapula against the chest wall; while, acting with the other muscles controlling the shoulder girdle, it gives a base on which the arm can move accurately. Loss of its nerve supply, the lateral thoracic nerve (C5–C7), allows the scapula to fall away from the chest wall, i.e. a 'winged scapula'. The muscle is used for most powerful forward movement of the arms. As the lower four to five of the digitations go to the inferior angle of the scapula, it also has an upward rotating action (**Figure 79**).

    Pectoralis minor is a protractor of the shoulder girdle. Running from the third, fourth and fifth ribs to the coracoid process, it also depresses the shoulder. It runs in the anterior wall of the axilla, behind the clavicular part of pectoralis major with which it usually works. As pectoralis major acts upon the

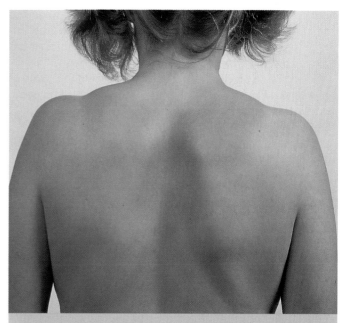

Figure 77 Elevation of the left shoulder is brought about by the upper fibres of trapezius and levator scapulae. The bulge caused by contracting trapezius is obvious, masking that in the underlying levator scapulae. In paralysis of trapezius, as after classical block dissection of the neck, levator scapulae then produces a very prominent ridge. Note that the lower fibres of trapezius are inactive, giving a hollow between the lower parts of the scapulae.

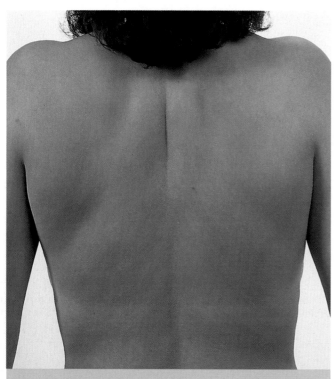

Figure 78 Retraction of the scapulae.

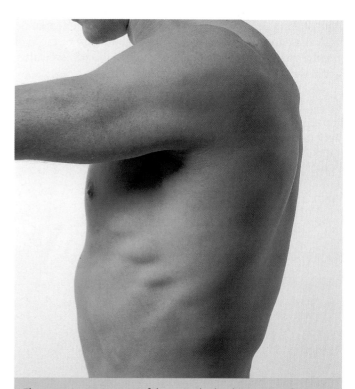

Figure 79 In protraction of the scapula the digitations of serratus anterior are obvious over the ribs.

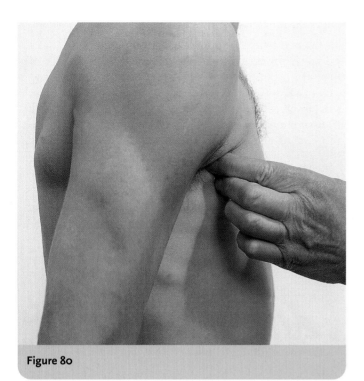

Figure 80

humerus, it can be inactivated by allowing the arm to hang freely at the side as the shoulder is protracted, when pectoralis minor can be felt contracting alone (**Figure 80**). It is supplied by the medial pectoral nerve (C8,T1).

MUSCLES ACTING OVER THE SHOULDER GIRDLE AND JOINT

Pectoralis major is a wide, fan-shaped muscle with two separate parts: clavicular and sternocostal. These are usually visible in a male (**Figure 81**) but are masked by the breast in a female (**Figure 82**). The clavicular part runs from the medial third of the clavicle, downwards and laterally to the crest of the greater tuberosity of the humerus (lateral lip of the bicipital groove). The sternocostal portion comes from two to six costal cartilages and related sternum. These fibres run upwards and laterally, deep to the clavicular portion, the lowest fibres going highest, increasing their downward pull on the humerus.

The whole muscle carries the arm forwards. The clavicular part elevates it, while the sternocostal fibres are powerful flexor-adductors. These fibres have a strong downward dislocating effect on the shoulder joint, which is balanced by the weak flexor-adductor but strong joint relocator, **coracobrachialis**. If the arms are fixed, the sternocostal fibres can be used as

1 Deltoid
2 Deltopectoral groove
3 Clavicular fibres of pectoralis major
4 Sternocostal fibres of pectoralis major

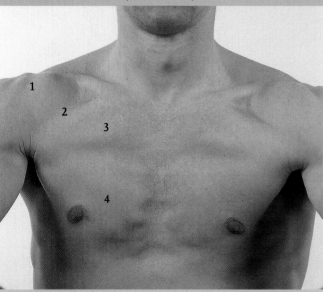

Figure 81 Action can be seen in the whole of pectoralis major when pressing the hands together across the chest, both parts of the muscle being easily identified. The lower fibres curve up deep to the clavicular, giving the anterior wall to the axilla, with pectoralis minor behind them and the anterior fibres of deltoid overlapping.

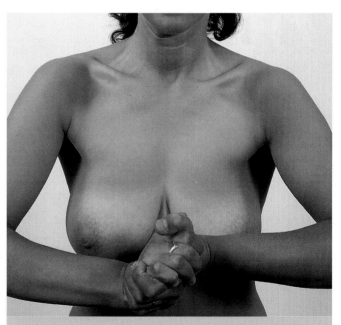

Figure 82 In a female much of pectoralis major is overlapped by the breast, limiting direct observation to the upper part: the clavicular portion is visible, with the confluence of the muscle to the axilla. Even here the axillary tail of the breast overlaps the lowest part.

accessory inspiratory muscles, as in respiratory distress (dyspnoea) due to disease or after severe exercise (**Figure 83**).

The upper part of the muscle is innervated by the lateral pectoral nerve (C5–C7) and the lower by the medial pectoral nerve (C8,T1).

Latissimus dorsi (Figure 84) covers much of the back below trapezius. It is attached to the spines of the lower six thoracic vertebrae (beneath trapezius), the spines of the lumbar and sacral vertebrae by an aponeurotic lumbar fascia (overlying the erector spinae muscles), and the posterior part of the iliac crest. The muscle fibres converge to a ribbon-like tendon, running in the posterior wall of the axilla to the floor of the bicipital groove of the humerus, in front of teres major. It is a powerful adductor-extensor of the arm at the shoulder joint, secondarily depressing the shoulder girdle. Its powerful downward pull on the humerus could dislocate the shoulder joint but for synergistic muscles, primarily the **long head of triceps**. Both muscles can be seen acting in downward pressure by the arm (**Figure 84**).

It is supplied by the lateral thoracic nerve (C6–C8). This, like the nerve supplying serratus anterior, runs down the lateral wall of the chest, where it is vulnerable to injury. This may occur during surgical removal of the breast, while excising its axillary tail and lymph nodes. Functional loss of the muscle is not severe, therefore it is often used as a myocutaneous flap for tissue replacement, as is pectoralis major.

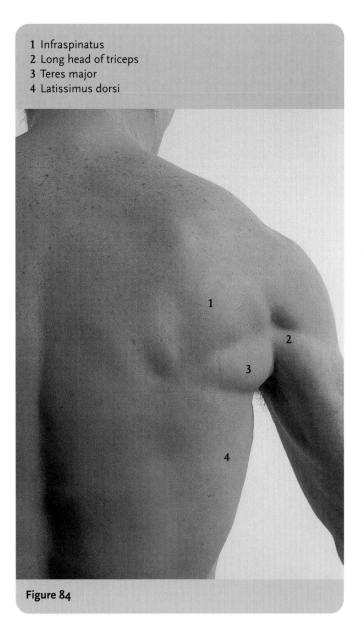

1 Infraspinatus
2 Long head of triceps
3 Teres major
4 Latissimus dorsi

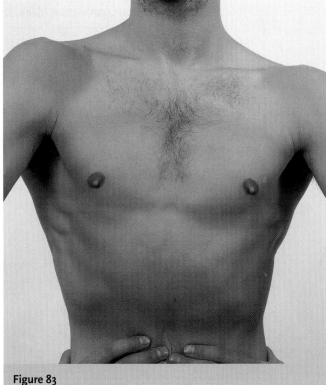

Figure 83

Figure 84

MUSCLES ACTING OVER THE SHOULDER JOINT

These are of two types: the rotator cuff muscles—whose tendons run through the capsule of the joint, acting also as dynamic ligaments—and the others. The **rotator cuff muscles** are supraspinatus (although not a rotator), subscapularis, infraspinatus and teres minor. Teres major, deltoid, coracobrachialis, biceps and the long head of triceps pass over the joint capsule. The close involvement of the rotator cuff muscles with the capsule of the joint reduces the need for other major ligaments, providing intrinsic stability as well as dynamic activity. However, even minor damage to any of these muscles or tendons can have quite severe effects on the fine neuromuscular control of the joint. **Supraspinatus** arises from the supraspinous fossa of the scapula, its tendon running through the capsule of the shoulder joint into the uppermost part of the greater tuberosity of the humerus. Because it is overlaid by trapezius, examination depends upon its function. It is an abductor of the arm, with its greatest value being in the first 15–20° of movement from the side, when deltoid is ineffective. In loss of its activity or its nerve—suprascapular nerve (C5–C6)—the arm can only be abducted actively if it can be swung out (**Figure 85**) or lifted to where deltoid becomes effective.

Deltoid is the other major abductor. Arising from the lateral third of the clavicle, the acromion and the underside of the spine of the scapula, the fibres cover the shoulder joint to converge onto the lateral aspect of the humerus (**Figure 73**). Its anterior fibres also act in flexion and medial rotation, while the posterior fibres support extension and lateral rotation. It is supplied by the **axillary nerve** (C5–C6), which, running round the neck of the humerus, is vulnerable in fractures of the neck of the bone and dislocations of the shoulder joint (see page 75).

Subscapularis is not available for direct examination. Coming from the deep surface of the scapula, its tendon runs through the joint capsule to the lesser tuberosity of the humerus. It is a powerful medial rotator of the humerus at the shoulder joint and its loss (or its nerve, C5–C6) makes it difficult to pass the hand behind the back (see **Figure 98b, and page 49**).

Teres major is a medial rotator and adductor, with some extension. Unlike subscapularis, it can easily be seen in activity when the arm is rotated medially, where it forms the greater part of the posterior wall of the axilla (**Figures 84 and 86**, left arm).

Infraspinatus and teres minor are both lateral rotators. Infraspinatus comes from the infraspinous fossa of the scapula; teres minor, alongside it, from the axillary border. They run to the greater tuberosity of the humerus, both usually being visible on forced external rotation (**Figure 86**, right arm).

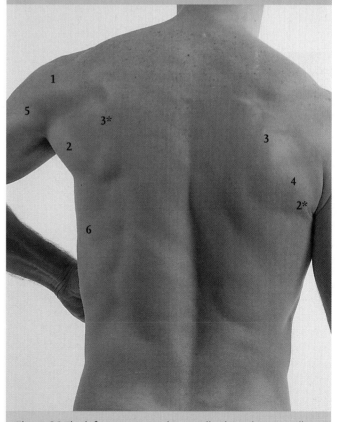

1   Deltoid
2   Teres major active
2*   Teres major relaxed
3   Infraspinatus active
3*   Infraspinatus relaxed
4   Teres minor
5   Long head of triceps
6   Latissimus dorsi

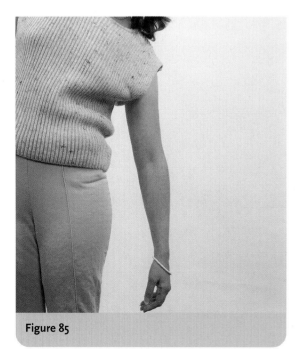

Figure 85

Figure 86 The left arm is rotated internally, the right externally.

1 Pectoralis major
2 Short head of biceps with coracobrachialis
3 Triceps
4 Teres major with the tendon of latissimus dorsi
5 Brachial vessels and plexus

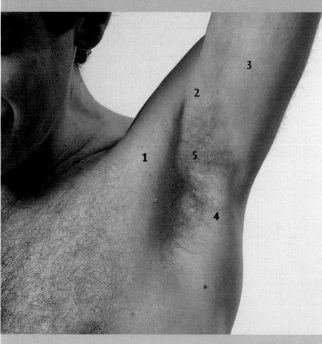

Figure 87

They have different nerve supplies: infraspinatus from the suprascapular branch of the brachial plexus (C5–C6); teres minor from the axillary nerve (C5–C6).

The **axilla** has an anterior wall of pectoralis major, with pectoralis minor behind it. The posterior wall is teres major, with the tendon of latissimus dorsi in front (**Figure 87**). Close to pectoralis major, the short head of biceps and coraco-brachialis run down the arm, with the cords of the brachial plexus and brachial vessels immediately behind. The axilla has important **lymph glands**, draining lymphatics from the arm and, most importantly, from the breast. The pulsations of the **axillary artery** can be felt against the humerus (**Figure 88**) and lower, as the brachial artery, in the groove to the medial side of biceps muscle.

The medial, lateral and posterior **cords of the brachial plexus** bear those relationships to the axillary artery. Pressure in the axilla can induce sensations of nerve compression and the nerves are also available for local anaesthetic block. However, as the cords are spread around the artery and the large vein(s), the technique is less easy than at the more prox-imal sites (see page 32).

Examination of the axilla is often required to elicit whether lymph glands are swollen and palpable, as from infection or carcinoma. Glands are in all parts of the axilla but, in cases of possible spread from the breast, particular care must be taken to examine the anterior wall behind pectoralis major (**Figure 89**).

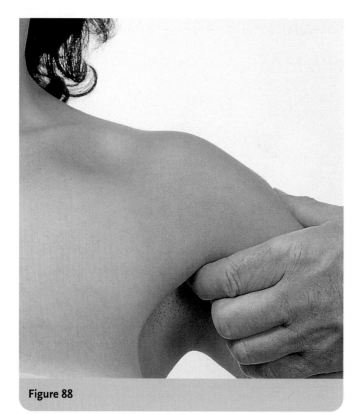

Figure 88

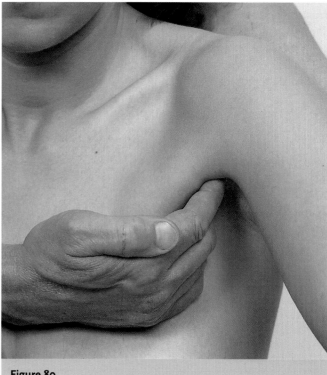

Figure 89

THE BONES OF THE ELBOW AND FOREARM

The humerus is surrounded by muscle but its epicondyles are palpable at the elbow (**Figure 90**). The **medial epicondyle** is the more prominent, though it is masked anteriorly by the common origin of the forearm flexor muscles. The ulnar nerve runs in a groove on its posterior aspect, where it is easily palpable and vulnerable (the so-called 'funny-bone'). The **lateral epicondyle** is also more easily palpated from behind, its anterior surface being masked by the common origin of the forearm extensor muscles.

The **olecranon of the ulna** gives the point to the elbow (**Figure 90**) and is the lever of insertion of triceps muscle. The olecranon and the epicondyles are level in the extended elbow but form a triangle in flexion (**Figure 91**), a relationship that may be changed in fractures around the region.

The **posterior border of the ulna** is palpable through to the prominent distal end or head at the wrist, with the styloid process at its tip (**Figure 92**).

The **head of the radius** should be palpable below the lateral epicondyle, particularly as the forearm is rotated, as should the joint space between it and the capitulum of the humerus (**Figure 93**). The lower half of the radius is palpable

1 Triceps
2 Brachioradialis
3 Extensor carpi radialis
4 Lateral epicondyle of humerus
5 Anconeus
6 Extensor muscles of forearm
7 Olecranon with overlying bursa
8 Ulnar nerve in cubital tunnel
9 Medial epicondyle of humerus
10 Flexor carpi ulnaris

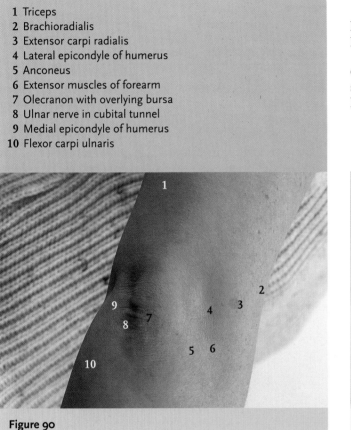

Figure 90

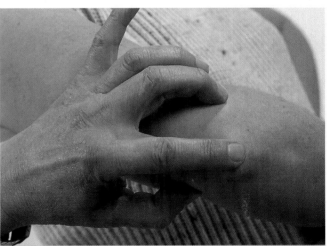

Figure 91 The thumb and middle finger overlay the epicondyles, the index finger the olecranon.

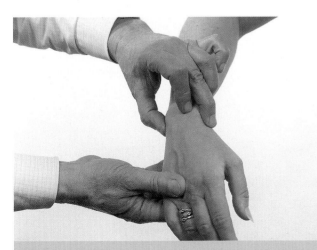

Figure 92 The examiner's thumb overlies the ulnar styloid, and the middle finger the radial styloid. The index indicates the radial tubercle.

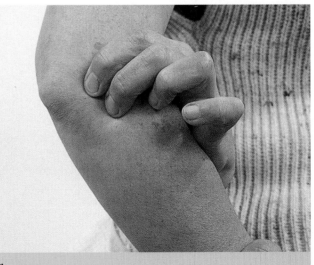

Figure 93

1 Tendon of extensor pollicis longus
2 Extensor pollicis brevis
3 Abductor pollicis longus
4 Radial styloid
5 Anatomical 'snuff-box'
6 Lunate

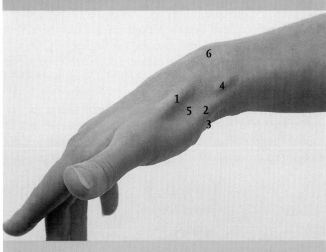

Figure 94

through to the radial styloid (**Figure 92**), which extends some 2 cm distal to that of the ulna. The dorsal tubercle of the radius (Lister's tubercle) is palpable on the back of the wrist (**Figure 92**). It is important to be aware of the feel and appearance of the distal end of the radius because of the common fractures of the region. **Abductor pollicis longus and extensor pollicis brevis** mask the tip of the **radial styloid process** on the border of the wrist, but it can be felt behind these tendons (**Figure 94**) and also anteriorly, where it produces a low swelling between the tendons of abductor pollicis longus and **flexor carpi radialis**.

MUSCLES OF THE UPPER ARM

Biceps brachii is the most prominent muscle in the region and isometric activity to 'show the muscle' is well known (**Figure 95**).

It arises by two heads. A long one comes from the supra-glenoid tubercle of the scapula, its tendon running through the shoulder joint (with a synovial sleeve) and then the inter-tubercular sulcus (bicipital groove). The short head arises, with coracobrachialis, from the coracoid process of the scapula and runs down medial to the long head. The two bellies join above

1 Deltoid
2 Biceps long head
3 Biceps short head with coracobrachialis
4 Triceps long head
5 Triceps medial head
6 Medial epicondyle of humerus
7 Brachialis
8 Medial intermuscular septum
9 Brachial artery with medial and ulnar nerve

1 Triceps
2 Biceps
3 Tendon of biceps
4 Bicipital aponeurosis
5 Brachialis

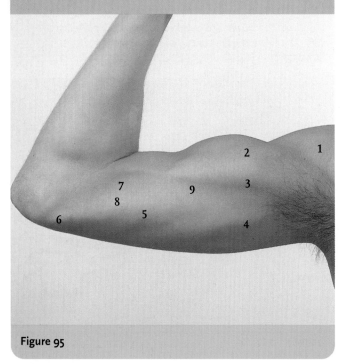

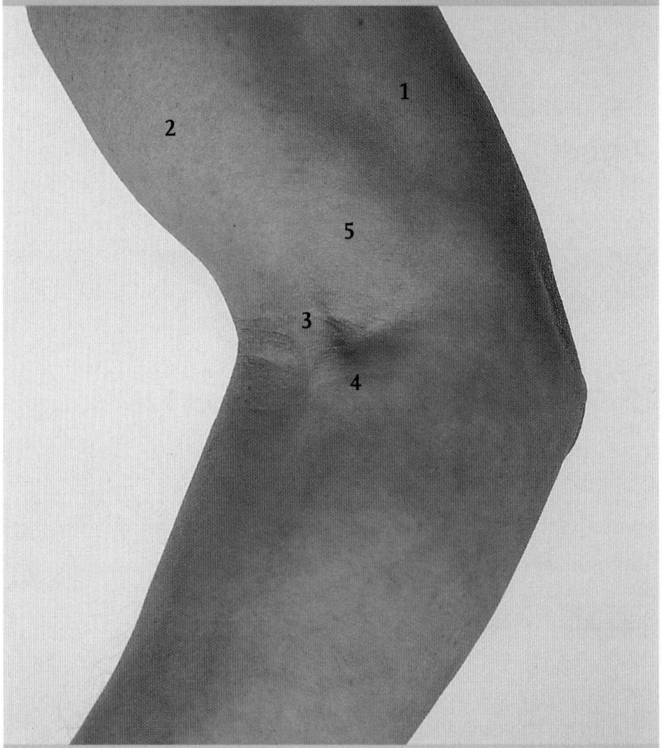

Figure 95

Figure 96

the elbow joint to form a tendon, inserted into the bicipital tuberosity of the radius. It is a powerful flexor at the elbow and supinator of the forearm. At the shoulder it is primarily a supporter of the joint. Close to the elbow a flat sheet runs medially from the main tendon, the bicipital aponeurosis, to be inserted, via the the deep fascia around the arm, into the ulna (**Figure 96**). This sheet, visible when under tension in supination, transmits flexor pull to the ulna. It also overlies and protects the main vessels and the median nerve at the elbow; the basilic vein, however, runs over it (see page 73).

Coracobrachialis runs deep to biceps for a variable distance down the arm and is inserted into the medial aspect of the humerus. It can be separated functionally from biceps by forcibly adducting the arm at the shoulder (i.e by pectoralis major) and with the elbow straight, with biceps relaxed.

Brachialis is a pure flexor at the elbow. It arises from the front of the humerus and runs down anterior to the elbow joint into the coronoid process of the ulna. Largely underlying biceps, it is less obvious from the surface, but it extends beyond biceps, particularly laterally (**Figures 96 and 97**).

All three muscles are supplied by the **musculocutaneous nerve** (C5–C7).

Triceps brachii (**Figures 95 and 97**) forms the bulk on the back of the arm, though the three heads can often be seen separately. The **long head** arises from the infraglenoid tubercle of the scapula, where it plays its main role in supporting the shoulder joint when the arm is loaded. The **lateral head** arises from the back of the humerus, above and lateral to the radial groove (**Figure 97**), while the **medial head** (**Figure 95**) comes from below and medial to the groove. The lateral and long heads join together and overlie the medial head as they approach their common insertion into the olecranon (**Figure 90**).

Triceps is the main extensor at the elbow joint. The **radial nerve**, the terminal branch of the posterior cord of the brachial plexus (C5–C8 and T1), runs around the shaft of the humerus, in the radial groove, deep to triceps and supplying it. Fractures to the midshaft of the humerus often lead to damage to the radial nerve; however, as the branches to triceps leave above this level, they are usually spared, and with them triceps (and anconeus).

1 Deltoid
2 Biceps
3 Brachialis
4 Long head of triceps
5 Lateral head of triceps
6 Lateral epicondyle of humerus
7 Olecranon

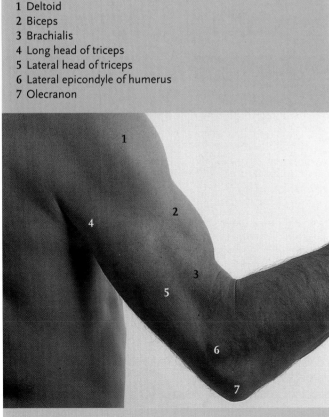

Figure 97

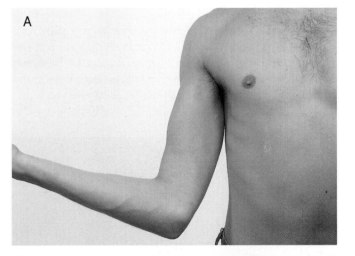

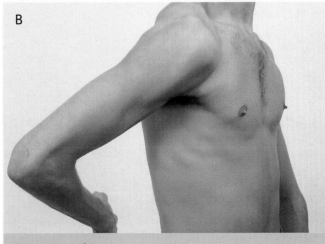

Figure 98A and B

THE FOREARM

The elbow joint is often considered to be a pure hinge joint. Lateral movement at the elbow joint proper is minimal, limited by the collateral ligaments and their supporting muscles (the extensor and flexor groups of the forearm). However, during pronation and supination, some lateral movement of the ulna is essential at the elbow joint (**Figure 100**). Failure to appreciate this leads to disastrous failures of pure flexor elbow prostheses.

The line of the arm through the elbow to the forearm in the supine (anatomical) position has a lateral angulation of some 10–20°, particularly in women; but this, the so-called carrying angle, is lost in the mid-prone position used for normal carriage.

Rotation in the arm occurs at the shoulder joint and, as pronation and supination, in the forearm. With the arm extended at the elbow, both can effect the direction of the hand; therefore, in this position, failure at one site can be overcome to some extent. With the arm flexed at the elbow, the two functions become separated, so clinical examination of the two joint systems should be done with the elbow flexed.

At the shoulder, the direction of the forearm can be used as the register of rotation. External rotation should allow some 90°, i.e. into the plane of the trunk (**Figure 98A**), while internal rotation should allow the forearm to be brought across the front of the body or placed behind the back (**Figure 98B**). As a quick and useful clinical guide to functional rotation at the shoulder, the patient can be asked if they can attend to their own hair and (if a woman) can fasten their brassiere straps at the back or (in both sexes) if they can touch the opposite scapula.

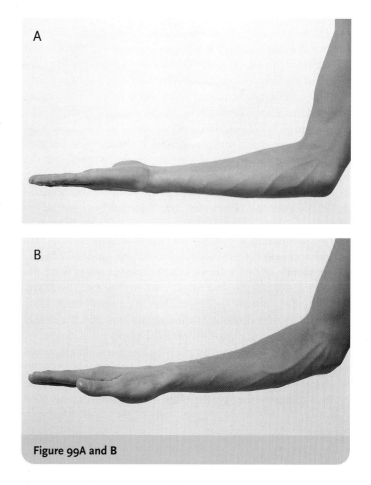

Figure 99A and B

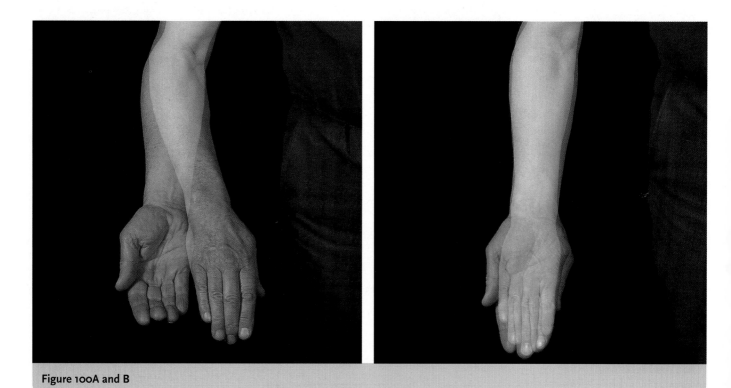

Figure 100A and B

Test pronation and supination with the elbow flexed and at the side. The palm of the hand should be able to face upwards and possibly a little outwards in supination (**Figure 99A**) and to be placed comfortably onto a flat surface in pronation (**Figure 99B**).

Pronation and supination are extremely valuable movements and any loss is a major disability. The movement is brought about by rotation of the forearm bones around an axis through the head of the radius to the attachment of the triangular fibrocartilage of the distal radio-ulnar joint to the base of the ulnar styloid. However, the distal end of the radius does not move around a fixed ulna. Were that so, the hand would flap around that fixed point and would be useless for rotatory activity (**Figure 100A**). The hand must be carried on a **functional** axis from the head of the radius through the distal end of the radius, lunate and capitate bones of the wrist; thence to the index, and middle metacarpals and fingers. To achieve this, the ulna must move laterally at the elbow to produce a reciprocal movement to that of the radius at the distal radio-ulnar joint (**Figure 100B**).

The cubital fossa is the hollow on the front of the elbow (**Figure 101**). The medial wall is made up of the common flexor muscles from the medial epicondyle of the humerus, particularly pronator teres, with brachioradialis forming the lateral wall. With both pronator teres and brachioradialis being inserted into the radius, the fossa is triangular. Its floor is the muscle and tendon of brachialis, with contributions from the capsule of the elbow joint and from supinator over the radius. It contains, or is overlaid by, several important vascular and nervous structures (see pages 73 and 76).

Brachioradialis muscle (**Figure 101**), running from the lateral supracondylar ridge of the humerus to the radius, is an important flexor muscle at the elbow joint, operating most efficiently with the forearm in the mid-prone position. Being innervated by the radial nerve, it can give good flexor power if the more proximal flexors lose their musculocutaneous nerve supply.

Pronator teres (**Figure 101**) comes from the medial supracondylar ridge and from the coronoid process of the ulna, running across to the outermost aspect of the curve of the radius. It is an important forearm pronator and a flexor at the elbow joint, particularly in pronation, when biceps is less effective. Being supplied by the median nerve, it can also be valuable as a flexor in loss of the musculocutaneous nerve.

Supinator lies in the floor of the cubital fossa, as it wraps around the radius from its posterior origin from the ulna. Innervated from the radial nerve by its posterior interosseous branch, it is a pure supinator of the forearm.

MOVEMENTS AT THE WRIST

The wrist joint strictly means the radiocarpal joint; however, as it always works with the midcarpal joints, they must be considered together—functionally and clinically—as the wrist. The wrist is capable of flexion, extension, abduction, adduction and circumduction. Flexion and extension are often considered the most important movements, even clinically. However, functionally, adduction (ulnar deviation) is by far the most important movement, with abduction (radial deviation) for recovery (**Figure 102**). A degree of ulnar deviation at the wrist is needed as the starting point for much normal posture and movement. It is the position for gripping most tools and household implements, e.g. knives, screwdriver, door handles etc., which must be in line with the forearm to allow for rotation. More dynamically, the plane of ulnar-radial movement is that required for use of a light hammer (**Figure 103**) or paint brush, or for controlling a chisel. A degree of flexion is useful, particularly for toiletry, whereas a little fixed extension gives maximal power to a hand grip. The range of ulnar deviation must be far greater than that of radial deviation, with greater precision of control (**Figures 104 and 105**).

Movement at the wrist is valuable, but even more so is its stability. The long muscles controlling the fingers cannot work effectively unless the wrist can be fixed. Conversely, if the wrist is to be moved under fine control, the fingers will almost always be fixed, as in a grip. When movement occurs at both sites, it will usually be in different planes, e.g. digital flexion with ulnar deviation at the wrist.

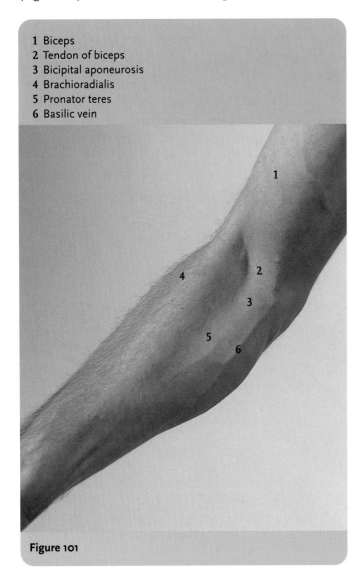

1 Biceps
2 Tendon of biceps
3 Bicipital aponeurosis
4 Brachioradialis
5 Pronator teres
6 Basilic vein

Figure 101

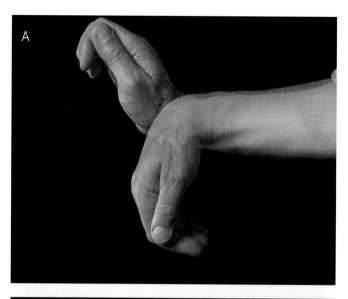

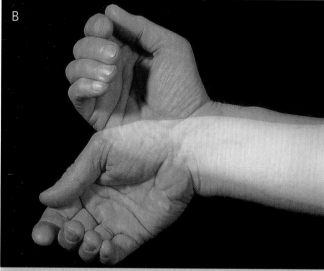

Figure 102A and B. Ranges of flexion and extention (A) Adduction and abduction (B).

Instability at the wrist leads to poor digital control, to improve which the wrist may need to be fixed by arthrodesis. Loss of joint movement can be largely overcome if the wrist is set in a degree of ulnar deviation, to allow objects to be gripped in line with the forearm. As many actions are carried out in the mid-prone position of the forearm, e.g. light

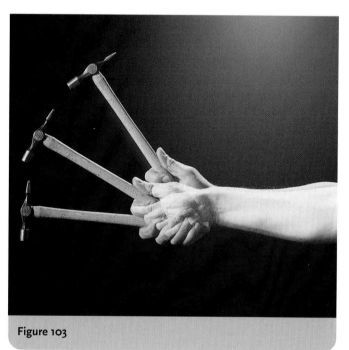

Figure 103

1 Radius	7 Trapezium
2 Ulna	8 Trapezoid
3 Scaphoid	9 Capitate
4 Lunate	10 Hamate
5 Triquetrum	11 Hook of hamate
6 Pisiform	

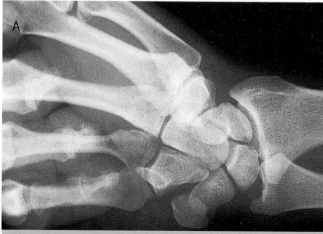

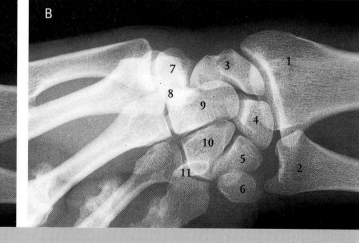

Figure 104A and B

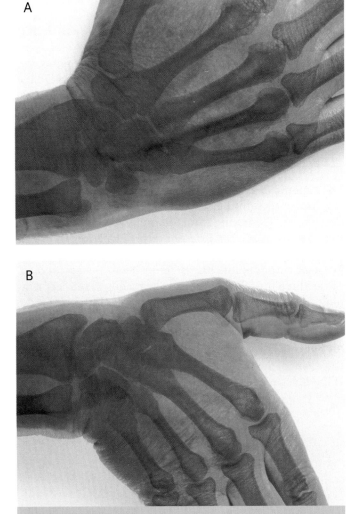

A

B

Figure 105A and B. Radial deviation (abduction, A) and ulnar deviation (adduction, B).

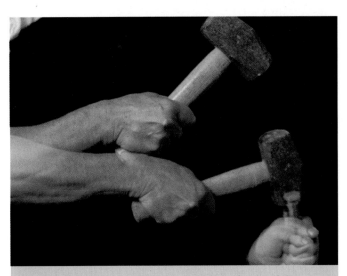

Figure 106 With a heavy hammer the wrist is fixed and the movement is essentially at the elbow.

hammering, these actions can be taken over by elbow activity which works in the same plane. In fact, under normal circumstances, the wrist is used for precision work, with the elbow taking over for heavier activities (**Figure 106**).

MUSCLES ON THE FRONT OF THE FOREARM

All the superficial muscles, with the exception of brachialis (see page 49) arise from the medial epicondyle of the humerus (above in the case of **pronator teres**, see page 51). **Palmaris longus** and **flexor carpi radialis** arise only from the epicondyle, and run superficially down the forearm, palmaris longus centrally and flexor carpi radialis more to the radial side, their tendons being prominent at the wrist. **Flexor digitorum superficialis** arises also from the coronoid process of the ulna and the oblique line of the radius; its tendons form a fullness to the ulnar side of palmaris longus. **Flexor carpi ulnaris** arises additionally from the posterior border of the ulna, by tendinous fibres that arch over the ulnar nerve (fibres that frequently lead to compression of the nerve), and runs down the ulnar border of the forearm to the pisiform and through this bone, by ligaments, to the hook of the hamate and fifth metacarpal.

Flexor carpi ulnaris is supplied by the ulnar nerve (C7–C8), whereas the other muscles receive their supply from the median nerve.

Deep to these muscles are **flexor digitorum profundus and flexor pollicis longus**. Although vital in the power flexor control of the digits, they are not readily seen from the surface in the forearm; while deeper still, **pronator quadratus** crosses between the radius and ulna in the distal quarter of the forearm. All three muscles receive innervation from the median nerve, though the parts of flexor digitorum to the ring and little fingers are supplied by the ulnar nerve.

TENDONS ON THE FRONT OF THE WRIST

On firm or resisted flexion at the wrist, palmaris longus (if present) and flexor carpi radialis are very prominent (**Figure 107**).

Palmaris longus, although only small, is quite a powerful flexor at the wrist, its superficial insertion into the flexor retinaculum giving it excellent leverage. However, it is often absent (13% of cases) and variable in form. Its tendon is often used as a tendon graft. When it is absent, the tendons of flexor digitorum superficialis become more prominent, particularly that to the index finger, which may be confused by the unwariness of that of palmaris longus.

The **flexor carpi radialis** tendon lies along the axis of radiocarpal movement and hence flexor control. It is often called an abductor at the wrist, an untenable description. It is a pure flexor but, being bound into its own tunnel close to the carpus, acts with its counterpart **extensor carpi radialis brevis** to produce close compaction of the wrist, giving central stability of the joints.

The **flexor carpi ulnaris** tendon lies to the ulnar border of the wrist. Its insertion into the pisiform and thence through this bone, as the pisohamate and pisometacarpal ligaments

1 Flexor carpi radialis
2 Palmaris longus
3 Flexor digitorum superficialis
4 Flexor carpi ulnaris
5 Abductor pollicis longus
6 Radial styloid
7 Pisiform with palmaris brevis

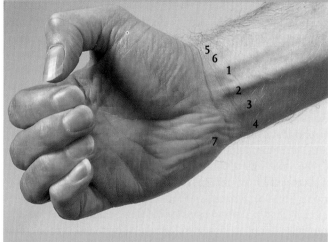

Figure 107 Tendons on the front of the wrist.

gives it excellent leverage for flexion, while acting with its extensor counterpart gives strong ulnar deviation on the radio-carpal base. The muscle is, in fact, of prime importance in most of the dynamic activity at the wrist.

Flexor digitorum superficialis, with the deeper **flexor digitorum profundus and flexor pollicis longus**, run through the **carpal tunnel**, formed from the curved carpus with the overlying **flexor retinaculum** (page 70).

MUSCLES ON THE BACK OF THE FOREARM

The superficial extensor muscles arise from the lateral epicondyle of the humerus and the supracondylar ridge. Brachioradialis, arising from the ridge, has been described (see page 51), as a flexor. **Extensor carpi radialis longus** comes from the supracondylar ridge, below brachioradialis, while **extensor carpi radialis brevis** comes from the epicondyle. These three muscles can usually be readily identified, running down the radial aspect of the forearm (**Figure 108**).

Extensor digitorum (communis) comes from the common extensor origin and forms a longitudinal swelling along the back of the forearm, running to the centre of the wrist. Extension of the individual fingers shows marked separation of the muscle into its digital components (**Figure 109**).

1 Brachioradialis
2 Extensor carpi radialis longus
3 Extensor carpi radialis brevis
4 Extensor digitorum
5 Extensor carpi ulnaris

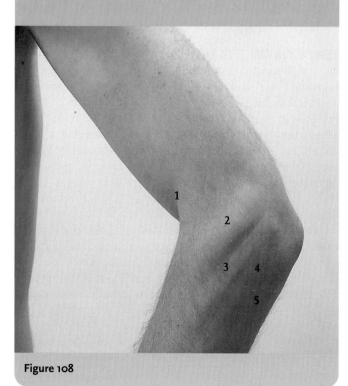

Figure 108

1 Extensor carpi radialis longus
2 Extensor carpi radialis brevis
3 Extensor digitorum
4 Extensor carpi ulnaris<None>
5 Subcutanrios border of ulna
6 Abductor pollicis longus

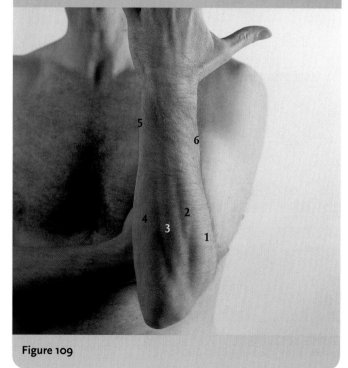

Figure 109

Extensor carpi ulnaris lies between extensor digitorum and the subcutaneous surface of the ulna, forming a prominent swelling when the wrist is tensed or, particularly, when the ulnar is deviated (**Figure 109**). The small **extensor digiti minimi** lies between the two above-mentioned muscles but, from the surface, is difficult to differentiate from the extensor digitorum component to the little finger.

Anconeus runs from the lateral epicondyle across to the ulna. It becomes prominent from the surface in pronation, when it pulls the ulna across and behind the radius.

Anconeus, brachioradialis and extensor carpi radialis longus are supplied by the radial nerve; the other extensor muscles, by its posterior interosseous branch.

TENDONS ON THE BACK OF THE WRIST

The flexor tendons are concentrated in relation to the carpal tunnel, whereas the extensors are spread around the outside of the bony carpal arch, the extensor retinaculum having six fibro-osseous compartments over the distal aspects of the radius and ulna.

Abductor pollicis longus, usually with two (even three) tendons, runs over the radial styloid in the same compartment as the more dorsally placed **extensor pollicis brevis** (**Figure 110A**). As the latter tendon may be absent or very small, it is important, surgically, to be aware of the likely reduplication of the abductor tendons.

The second compartment transmits the two **extensor carpi radialis** tendons (**Figure 110B**), longus going to the base of the second metacarpal, and brevis to the third. **Extensor pollicis longus** crosses these two tendons, turning around the dorsal (Lister's) tubercle of the radius, and runs to the distal phalanx of the thumb. When the thumb is extended, the raised tensed thumb tendons create a hollow between them, the '**anatomical snuff-box**', with the scaphoid and trapezius in its base (**Figure 110A**). Owing to the overlying tendon, the two carpi radialis tendons are less easy to examine. If the wrist is forcibly extended against resistance, with the thumb flexed, the tendon of extensor carpi radialis can be felt just distal to the end of the radius and the brevis tendon before its insertion. As the radialis longus muscle acts with abductor pollicis longus in radial deviation of the wrist, this movement resisted, with the thumb flexed, will make these two tendons obvious (**Figure 110B**).

Tendons of **extensors digitorum and indicis** run together through the fourth compartment, still over the dorsal surface of the radius, while the small **extensor digiti minimi** tendon runs in the fifth, over the radio-ulnar joint (**Figure 110B**).

Extensor carpi ulnaris runs over the dorsum of the ulna **only in full supination**. With movement towards pronation, including the main functional mid-prone position, the tendon runs on the ulnar border of the wrist, where it can be felt, on forced ulnar deviation, running in the gap between the ulnar styloid and the base of the fifth metacarpal. This fact is very little appreciated. In rheumatoid arthritis, where there is increased dorsal movement of the distal end of the ulna, operations have often been performed to return the tendon to what was erroneously thought to be its correct position.

1 Abductor pollicis longus	5 Extensor carpi radialis longus
2 Extensor pollicis brevis	6 Extensor digitorum with indicis
3 Cephalic vein	7 Extensor digiti minimi
4 Extensor pollicis longus	

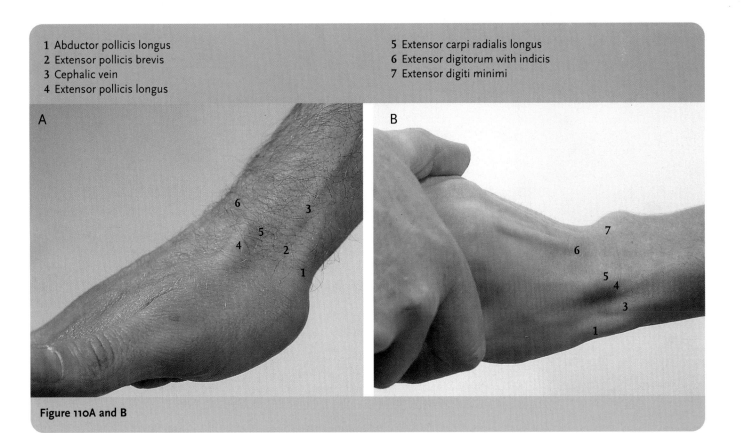

Figure 110A and B

Chapter 5

The hand

The hands exhibit remarkable mechanical functions, possible only through a very great sensory input. The hand's efficiency depends upon its remarkable neurological control, with its large cortical representation in the brain.

The hands exhibit a most important **epicritic sensory** function. The hairless skin of the palm develops from an embryonic special sensory placode into the area of special tactile sensibility. This area is present—and most valuable—even at the tip of a congenital 'amputated' limb, making it a much more useful instrument than one after a traumatic amputation. A congenital amputee will often use the available limb tip, to utilise its special sensibility where possible, in preference to the variety of prostheses preferred by the traumatic amputee.

The **epicritic sensibility of the palm** offers sensory perception not available from skin elsewhere, while fine sensory input also permits the hand's exquisite mechanical control. The hand has been described as 'the eyes that see in the dark and around corners'. The correct coin can be taken from a pocket or bag simply by touch; by developing the necessary additional sensory awareness, it can be used to read Braille (**Figure 111**); it can assemble equipment, nuts, bolts, etc., in positions where direct vision is impossible. These activities could not be carried out with the normal tactile sensibility available to other parts of the body, or in a hand after median nerve section. Even with ideal repair, there will be fewer available nerve fibres; however, perception training, sadly often neglected, can be of great help in making maximal use of those available.

The skin on the back of the hand must be quite loose to permit the range of movement; full flexion increases the skin distance from wrist to fingertip by some 30%. In the fingers, although adherent over the middle and distal phalanges, surplus skin is provided at the joints, producing the transverse ridging (**Figure 112**). The dorsal skin is elastic and shows normal body pigmentation.

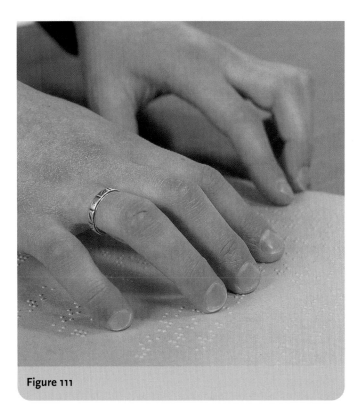

Figure 111

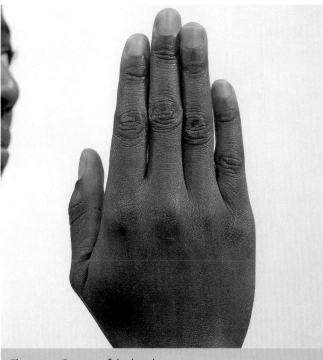

Figure 112 Creases of the hand.

The **palmar skin** is quite different. Even in dark-skinned races, the palm remains pale: only the flexion creases show full pigmentation (**Figure 113**). The hairless skin is thick and the surface thrown up into **papillary ridges**, beneath which are large numbers of sensory end-organs. The ridge pattern is characteristic for the individual and, while being of prime sensory function, the ridges are also set in a manner to assist grip (**Figure 114**). Over the palm the skin lacks sebaceous glands but has large numbers of sweat glands, which, in addition to thermoregulation, also keep the epidermis soft and supple. The palmar skin must be more fixed. It is bound to the palmar fascia in a central triangle and at the flexion creases. The intervening regions

have **fibro-fatty pressure pads**, important for grip. The pads at the fingertips are further specialised: the distal part is a firmly supported tactile zone, whereas the more proximal part is readily deformable for grip, the firmer distal part acting also as a stop pad (**Figure 115**).

The distal palmar pad and those of the proximal and middle phalanges overlie and are bound to transverse fibrous flexor sheaths, which act also as retinacular systems for the digital tendons. The distal digital pad is supported by fibrous binding to the terminal phalanx, but the nail also gives it considerable lateral and distal support. The nail-bearing area, i.e. beyond the dorsal distal flexion crease, has palmar innervation and the skin is hairless.

1 Distal wrist
2 Thenar
3 Proximal palmar
4 Distal palmar
5 Metacarpophalangeal
6 Proximal interphalangeal
7 Distal interphalangeal
8 Thumb interphalangeal

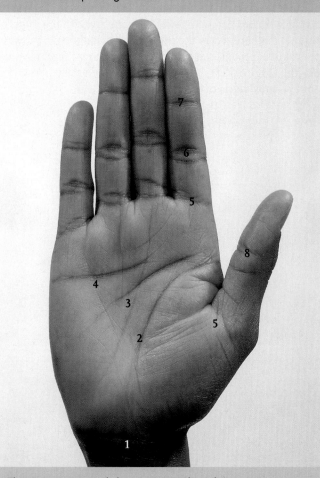

Figure 113 Pigmented skin creases in the palm.

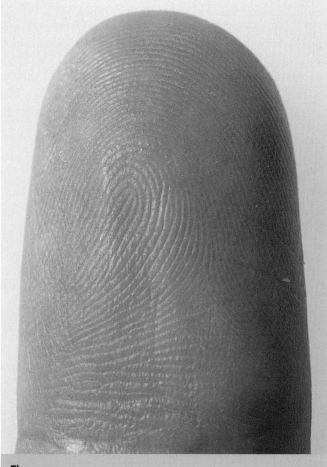

Figure 114

The nail (**Figure 116**) is made of hard keratin. A **nail groove** is formed on either side. Here the nail is attached to the epidermis at the **nail wall** and also where the **eponychium** overlies and is adherent to the root of the nail. Loss of adherence, both laterally and at the eponychium (often due to crude manicuring), exposes the region to infection, which commonly becomes chronic and difficult to cure. The **nail root** lies beneath the overlying skin proximal to the eponychium.

Between the bases of the fingers, the **palmar webs**, level with the proximal digital creases, extend some 1–2 cm beyond

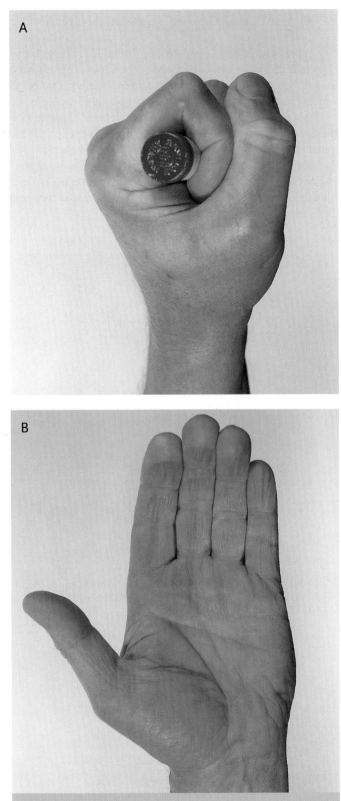

A

B

Figure 115A and B. The tube has been gripped firmly, showing the role of the pads in producing pressure on the object (**A**). The hand was photographed immediately after release of pressure, showing the areas of deformation (**B**). Note how the proximal part of the digital pad shows deformation, whereas the firmer tactile zone has remained as a stop pad.

1 Body of nail
2 Nail wall
3 Lateral nail groove
4 Lunula (best seen on thumb and index finger)
5 Eponychium
6 Nail bed in proximal nail groove
7 Approximate extent of nail bed

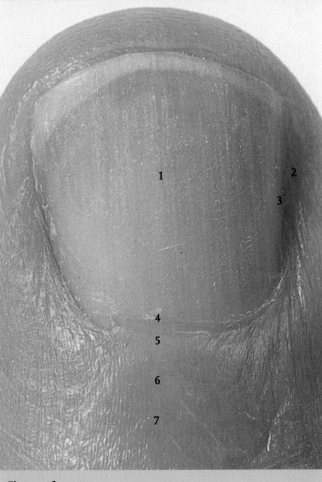

Figure 116

the **metacarpophalangeal joints** (Figure 117). The **distal palmar crease** is the actual crease for these joints and lies just proximal to them. The middle and distal digital creases are near to the **interphalangeal joints**. The palmar creases are lines of minimal tension and hence are ideal for surgical incisions (**Figure 118**).

At the **ulnar heel** of the palm, palmaris brevis pulls up the skin pad, increasing palmar contact in power grip; however, it also produces a protective pad over the ulnar nerve, which, although tucked in beside the pisiform bone, is vulnerable to external pressure, running, as it does, superficial to the flexor retinaculum.

BONY FEATURES OF THE CARPUS AND HAND

The hand is, in effect, mounted on the radius, through the **scaphoid** and **lunate**, the distal end of the ulna being well separated from the **triquetrum**, so as to allow the wide range of movement into ulnar deviation (see pages 52 and 53).

On the back, with the wrist straight, the bases of the **metacarpal bones** are more prominent than the carpals, which are at the base of a shallow transversely running gutter, deep to the extensor tendons. In flexion the **lunate** makes a visible central swelling, distal to the radius (see **Figure 94**, page 48), with the **triquetrum**, separated by a gap from the distal end of the ulna.

1 Proximal digital creases
2 Distal palmar crease
3 Proximal palmar crease
4 Thenar crease
5 Distal wrist crease
6 Proximal wrist crease
7 Proximal interphalangeal crease
8 Distal interphalangeal crease

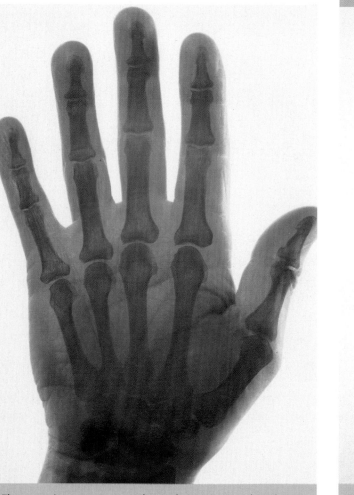

Figure 117 Anteroposterior radiograph superimposed on the hand.

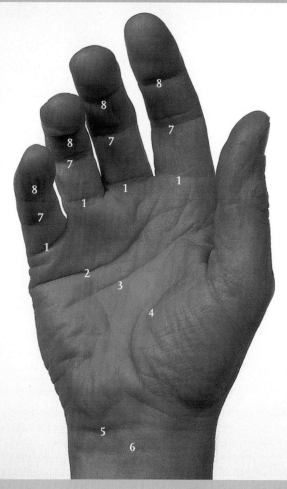

Figure 118

When the wrist is flexed, the transverse arch of the carpus is obvious from behind, forming the bony component of the carpal tunnel. Anteriorly, only the peripheral carpal bones can be felt. To the radial side, the **tubercle of the scaphoid** is palpable—and a swelling even visible—when the hand is in radial deviation (**Figure 119A**); surface pointers to its position are the tendon of flexor carpi radialis and the proximal end of the thenar crease of the palm. As the hand is carried into ulnar deviation the scaphoid becomes more in line with the distal end of the radius, so producing a hollow where the tubercle was (**Figure 119B**). The **tubercle of the trapezium** is less easy to feel, but is about 1 cm distal to that of the scaphoid (**Figure 120A**). The **pisiform** is prominent to the ulnar side, being the insertion of flexor carpi ulnaris, whereas the **hook of the hamate** is less easy to feel but still palpable by pressing about 1cm distal to the pisiform (**Figure 120B**). The **carpal ligament** (flexor retinaculum) crosses between these four points to produce the carpal tunnel (see pages 69 and 70).

The tubercles of the scaphoid and the pisiform are the bony resting points of the heel of the flat hand; hence the scaphoid's vulnerability to fracture when falling on the extended wrist. The scaphoid becomes trapped against the distal end of the radius,

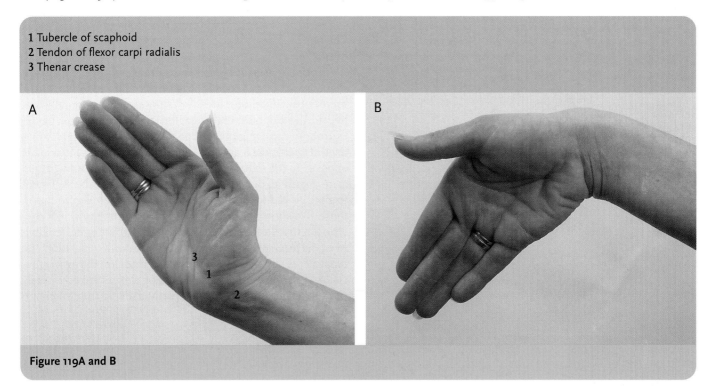

1 Tubercle of scaphoid
2 Tendon of flexor carpi radialis
3 Thenar crease

A

B

Figure 119A and B

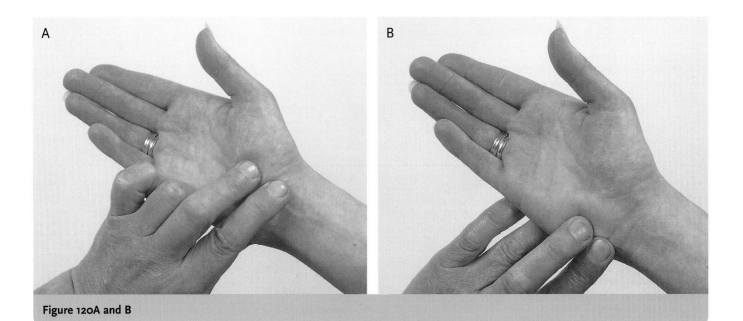

A

B

Figure 120A and B

whereas the pisiform is free to move and usually escapes injury. As the scaphoid (and the trapezium) lie in the base of the **anatomical snuff-box**, pain on pressure here, rather than over the tubercle, is characteristic of scaphoid fracture (**Figure 121**).

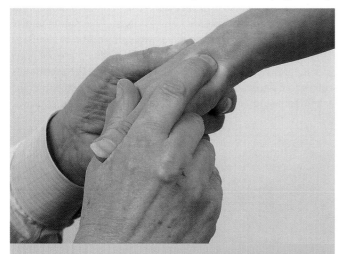

Figure 121 The finger is pressing over the scaphoid where pain is to be expected in scaphoid fracture.

A

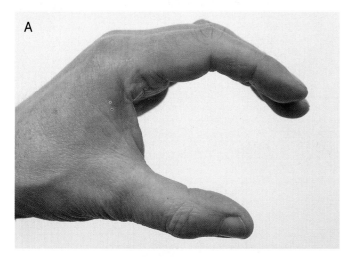

B

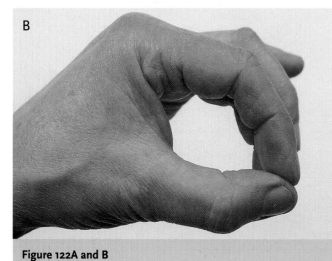

Figure 122A and B

The **metacarpals** and **phalanges** are all palpable dorsally throughout their length. The knuckles are made up of the heads of the bones at each joint. The **metacarpophalangeal joints** are readily palpable beyond the knuckles on the dorsum, particularly in flexion. The metacarpal heads project to the palmar side, overlaid by the deep transverse metacarpal ligament. They can be felt through the palmar pads, approximately level with the distal palmar crease for the index finger and a little beyond for the others.

HAND FUNCTIONS

The hand has two major functional patterns and several lesser ones.

Precision grip and finger movements require fine kinaesthetic control (and, usually, the fine tactile sensibility at the finger tips). To achieve precision, movement is normally limited to the digital metacarpophalangeal joints and, in the thumb, to the carpometacarpal joint, all other joints being fixed (**Figures 122A and B**). In the grip, the thumb is usually opposed to the index and middle fingers, to produce a 'tripod grip' (**Figure 123**). As thumb opposition may not be sufficient to give full pad-to-pad opposition to the fingers (**Figure 124A**), these also show a degree of rotation (**Figures 124B**). For precision activity, the median nerve controls the tactile sensibility of the three principal digits and also thumb opposition; the ulnar nerve supplies the interosseous muscles, the prime precision controls of the digits. The long flexors are essentially power flexors and are not normally used in fine precision

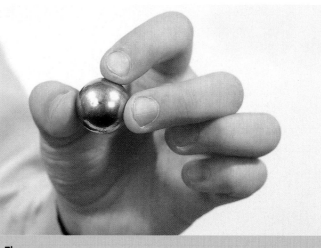

Figure 123

activity; they add power to the **pinch** or **flexion** where needed. Nevertheless, even the powerful-precision digital activities of a concert pianist come mainly from the highly trained interosseous muscles.

Power grip has the fingers flexed against the fixed thenar eminence, to produce an oblique grip at some 45° to the transverse axis of the hand. This obliquity is brought about by ulnar deviation and rotation of the digits at the metacarpophalangeal joints, together with flexion at the carpometacarpal joints of the ring and little fingers (**Figures 125A and B**). The thumb base, i.e. the metacarpal and the thenar pad, provides the fixed buttress, with the thumb often controlling the leverage of the object being gripped, or, if the object is large, the thumb assists by encircling. The hypothenar pad is pulled up by palmaris brevis to give palmar assistance (**Figure 126**). With this grip, together with ulnar deviation at the wrist, the object being held can be brought into line with the forearm for rotation (e.g. a screwdriver, door handle, etc.) or to achieve maximal effect from wrist or elbow movement (as in hammering etc.). The main power of digital flexion comes from the long flexor muscles, which are innervated by the median nerve, supplemented by the ulnar nerve to flexor digitorum profundus to the ring

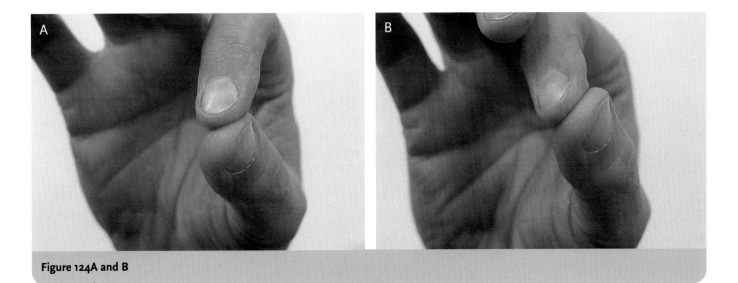

Figure 124A and B

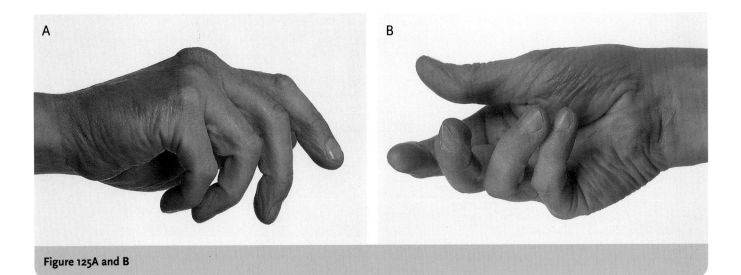

Figure 125A and B

and little fingers. The ulnar nerve is also responsible for control of the ulnar-sided interossei and the hypothenar muscles, to give the required digital opposition, as well as supplying flexor carpi ulnaris, the main ulnar deviator at the wrist. An oblique power grip therefore is impossible after loss of the ulnar nerve, which is responsible for transferring the not very useful transverse pure flexor grip of the hand (see *baggage grip*) into this most valuable oblique power grip, needed for so much manual activity.

Key or lateral pinch grip has the fingers held firmly together in flexion, with the thumb in partial opposition against the side of the index finger (**Figure 127**). The ulnar nerve innervation of the radial interossei, particularly the first dorsal, is needed, while the median nerve supplies thumb activity.

Hook or baggage grip is a simple transverse flexor grip or hooking of the fingers, used primarily in load bearing. Although both long flexors give full flexor power into the palm, for sustained loading, as in carrying baggage, flexor digitorum superficialis becomes predominant, i.e total median nerve innervation (**Figure 128**).

Power pinch is used on occasions but is essentially a precision-type grip with added long flexor activity (**Figure 129**). The interossei are often used to give digital deviation for screwing action. This grip becomes important in ulnar nerve palsy, when the oblique power grip becomes impossible.

Writing may be a little complicated to analyse; however, it can be reduced to finely controlled upstrokes of pure interosseous activity, giving metacarpophalangeal flexion and interphalangeal extension against the pen, with the long flexors being involved in downstrokes.

Development of grip

In early infancy the grip is essentially a transverse, long flexor muscle activity (**Figure 130**), producing a very efficient trans-

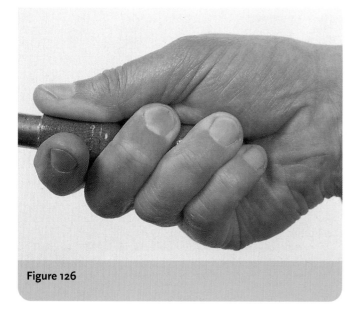

Figure 126

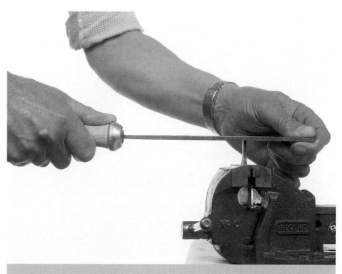

Figure 127 The handle of the file is controlled by a power grip and the tip by a key grip.

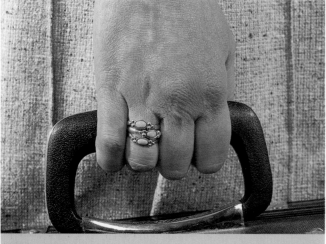

Figure 128

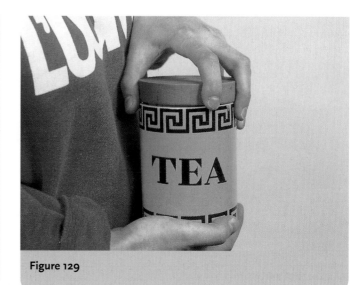

Figure 129

verse grip but without thumb opposition. Fine intrinsic and full sensory control must await the completion of myelination during the first 2 years of life.

MOVEMENTS OF THE FINGERS

The fingers should be able to flex into the palm, with their tips touching the proximal palmar crease. Any deficiency can be measured from the palm (**Figure 131**). The individual joints should produce 80–90° at the metacarpophalangeal joints (greater to the ulnar side); the proximal interphalangeal, 110° and the distal, 70–80°. Extension should be to 180° at all joints, though many people show a degree of hyperextension, particularly at the metacarpophalangeal joints. Any deficiency in extension can be measured from the line of the metacarpal. The distal interphalangeal joint allows some passive hyperextension to permit pad-to-pad opposition with the thumb.

The **interphalangeal joints** must have lateral stability and so show only flexion and extension.

The **metacarpophalangeal joints** additionally show lateral movement and some rotation; greatest in extension when the collateral ligaments are lax. As the fingers are flexed, the collateral ligaments tighten; at full flexion, free lateral movement is small, but the fingers are carried into a degree of ulnar deviation and rotation as is needed for a power grip. Abduction from the middle finger in extension is largely limited by tightness of the webs (see **Figure 141**, page 68). In the individual fingers, however, ulnar deviation is far greater than radial; by some three to four times in the index and middle fingers (**Figure 132**) and twice in the ring and little fingers. It is also a much more precise movement.

It is important that an inflamed hand is treated with all digital collateral ligaments taut, i.e. metacarpophalangeal joints flexed to 70° and the interphalangeal joints in full

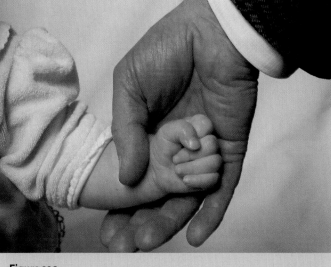

Figure 130

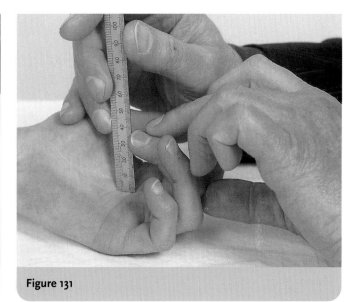

Figure 131

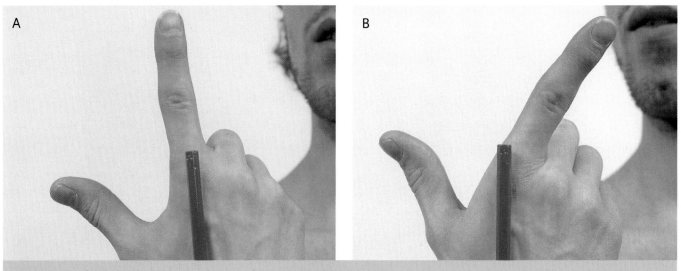

Figure 132A and B Radial deviation (**A**) and Ulnar deviation (**B**) of the finger.

extension, to prevent ligaments shortening (**Figure 133**). This can occur very rapidly, producing a fixed deformity. The so-called position of rest, so commonly practised, is **not** acceptable.

Thumb movements are complex. At the carpometacarpal joint, flexion, extension, abduction and adduction relative to the palm and opposition into the palm are described, but pure movements are virtually impossible. Ranges at the metacarpophalangeal joint vary with the individual, with flexion to some 60°, while hyperextension is common. Abduction and adduction are quite important, also being used to vary the position of thumb opposition to the individual fingers (**Figure 134**). When movement at the carpometacarpal joint is lost, as from arthrodesis, the range of movement at the metacarpophalangeal joint can partially compensate.

MUSCLES CONTROLLING THE DIGITS

Each finger has two long flexor tendons; flexor digitorum superficialis to the middle phalanx and profundus to the distal. **Flexor digitorum profundus** can be tested by the strength of a digital hook (**Figure 135**). Loss of **superficialis** may not be noticed except for some loss of flexor strength and, particularly, sustained power, as in baggage carrying. To test, the finger should be able to flex as the examiner holds the other fingers straight (**Figure 136**). NB Superficialis action on the little finger may be weak or even absent.

Flexor pollicis longus can be tested by hooking the thumb. A more general digital test can be to press the thumb pad to that of the little finger, resisting the examiner's pull (**Figure 137**), so also testing opposition and short-muscle activity in

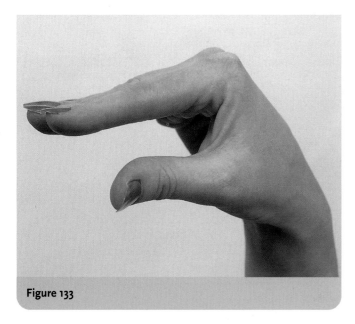

Figure 133

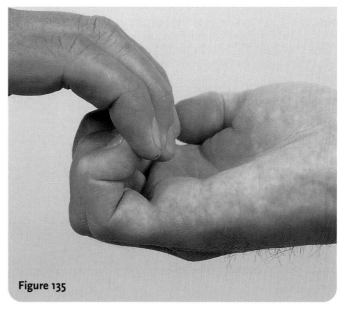

Figure 135

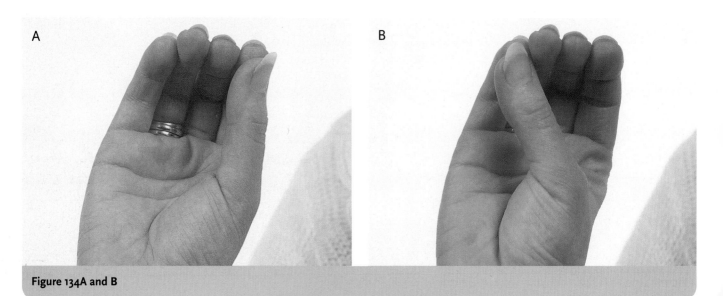

A

B

Figure 134A and B

the digits. Action in flexor carpi ulnaris should also be seen, fixing the pisiform and the hypothenar muscle origins.

Extensor digitorum communis presents some problems in that digital extension is linked with the actions of the interossei and lumbrical muscles, which can themselves extend the interphalangeal joints if there is some flexion at the metacarpophalangeal joints. Hence, although the long extensor is not directly linked to the proximal phalanx by a true tendon, the important test is the ability to extend the metacarpophalangeal joint. In the absence of the short muscles, the long muscle produces hyperextension at the metacarpophalangeal joints and will only extend the interphalangeal joints if the hyperextension is prevented. NB The index (extensor indicis) and little finger (extensor digiti minimi) have their additional long extensors, acting with extensor communis.

The thumb has a long extensor muscle over each joint, acts as an abductor at the carpo metacarpal joint of the thumb, but its major function is as a radial deviator at the wrist. **Extensor pollicis brevis** (often small or missing) acts over the metacarpophalangeal joint, with **extensor pollicis longus** running over the interphalangeal joint. All three tendons stand out in thumb extension, producing the 'anatomical snuff-box' (see page 55). As the extensor brevis also has an abductor pull, it does not show if the thumb is extended in adduction, a more direct line for the long muscle.

As is the case in the fingers, the intrinsic (here the thenar) muscles contribute to the extensor expansion, controlling interphalangeal extension. If the metacarpophalangeal joint is allowed to flex, then the interphalangeal joint can be extended, even in the absence of a long extensor (**Figure 138**).

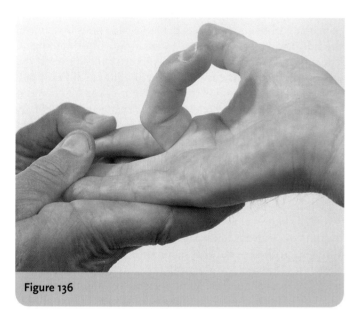

Figure 136

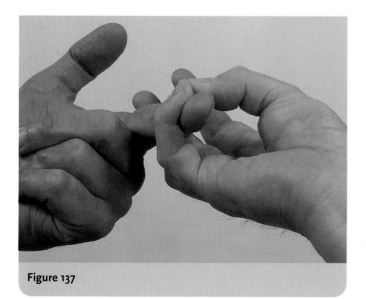

Figure 137

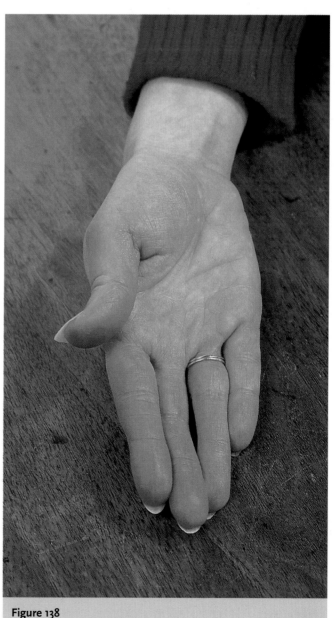

Figure 138

The main power then comes from adductor pollicis brevis, onto the distal part of the long extensor tendon (if intact), pulling to the medial side of the flexed metacarpophalangeal joint (see *Froment's sign*, **Figure 140**).

INTRINSIC MUSCLES

The thenar muscles are not easy to isolate from each other when testing, which is also complicated by their variable median and ulnar innervation. The **ulnar nerve** supplies **adductor pollicis brevis**, often the deep head of **flexor pollicis brevis**, and may contribute to **opponens**. The **median nerve** supplies **abductor pollicis brevis**, **opponens** and the superficial head of **flexor pollicis brevis**. The median nerve thus

produces opposition; however, if it is lost, ulnar nerve overlap into the deep head of the flexor and possibly opponens may help. **Abductor pollicis brevis**, commonly affected in carpal tunnel compression of the median nerve, can be tested by firm abduction of the thumb against resistance (**Figure 139**) (but, here, early electrodiagnostic tests are preferable, as recovery after nerve release is uncertain once muscle loss has occurred).

Flexor digitorum brevis activity can be tested by flexing at the metacarpophalangeal joint into the palm, whilst it also acts with **opponens** in forced opposition. It also acts with the abductor in forced abduction.

Adductor pollicis brevis can be tested by forcing the thumb against the side of the palm, but extensor pollicis longus also has an adductor pull in extension. **Froment's sign** is used as a specific test for the adductor muscle (**Figure 140**). A thin object, such as a strip of paper, is gripped between the pads of the thumbs and the sides of the proximal phalanges of the index fingers, keeping the interphalangeal joint of the thumb extended. As the hands are pulled apart, because the metacarpophalangeal joints are flexed, the long extensor is ineffective, the adductor being required to maintain interphalangeal extension. If the adductor is inactive, the thumb flexes at the interphalangeal joint due to the unopposed pull of flexor pollicis longus, as in the right hand of Figure 140.

The **interosseous muscles** are the primary (and particularly precision) flexors at the metacarpophalangeal joints of the fingers, through their attachment to the base of the proximal phalanges and their transverse fibres into the extensor expansion. By virtue of their wing tendons, they contribute to interphalangeal extension. In fine precision grip, this extensor component balances out the elastic pull of the two long flexors against the single long extensor, leaving the two interossei to the finger to combine to give metacarpophalangeal flexion, with each providing such ulnar or radial deviation as is required. To test their flexor role, the metacarpophalangeal joints should be flexed, with the interphalangeal joints extended. Traditionally, the

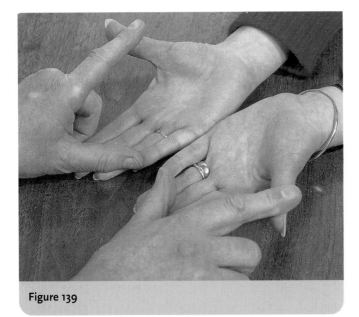

Figure 139

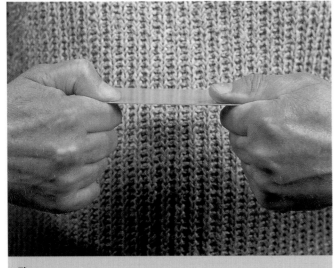

Figure 140

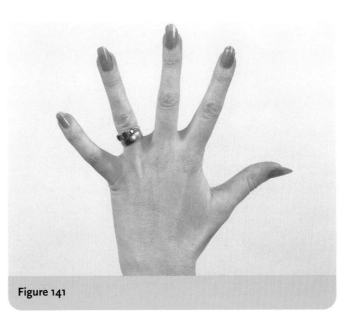

Figure 141

interossei have been divided morphologically into palmar adductors and dorsal abductors on the axis of the middle finger, with the result that the vital precision flexor role of these muscles is often neglected. Their abductor power can be tested by forced abduction of the fingers from the middle (**Figure 141**), whereas adduction can be examined by slipping a piece of paper between the extended fingers, the examiner pulling it out against adductor action (**Figure 142**).

The **lumbricals** are difficult to test. They act dynamically only in firm extension at the interphalangeal joints and, only then, can they flex the metacarpophalangeal joints. They can be seen in this role in limiting the clawing of the index and middle fingers in ulnar nerve palsy, when they are the only intrinsic muscles left to these fingers. In the normal hand this function is carried out by the interossei. It is now usually accepted that the lumbricals, with their rich sensory innervation, act as dynamic proprioceptive bridges between the flexor and extensor tendons. The **hypothenar** muscles act on the little finger essentially as ulnar-sided interossei but with added opponens function. They also form a dynamic continuum with flexor carpi ulnaris, which stabilises their origin on the pisiform and also acts as the carpometacarpal flexor.

DIGITAL VALUES

It is usual to think of the thumb as the most important digit because of its role in opposition, and in this the index and middle fingers play the primary role in the functional tripod. These digits also have the prime sensory functions. The little finger is often dismissed as of little importance but, in fact, it plays a vital role as a balance point of a functioning hand and, with its ulnar side having a most important sensory imput, indicates the relationship of the hand to an underlying surface (**Figure 143**). Other than for its important ring-bearing function for many people, the ring finger can be the most easily lost. Consequently, it is usually the digit of choice when a thumb replacement is required (pollicisation).

Retinaculi are vital in the hand to retain the tendons and to prevent bow-stringing across curves. This is particularly important in the fingers, where even a few millimetres of stretch in the retaining bands will reduce the range of digital flexion enormously.

At the wrist the **flexor retinaculum** is attached to the pisiform and the hook of the hamate on the ulnar side and to the tubercles of the scaphoid and trapezium on the radial (see page 61). It is some 3 cm in transverse length and some 4 cm distalwards, from the distal wrist crease to the level of the thenar

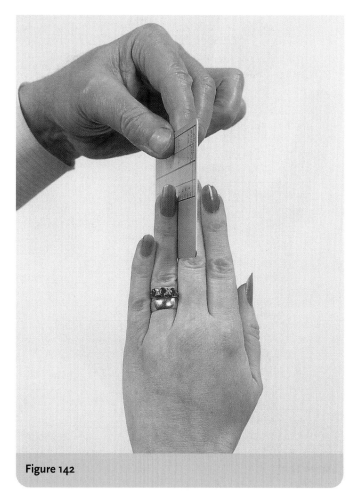

Figure 142

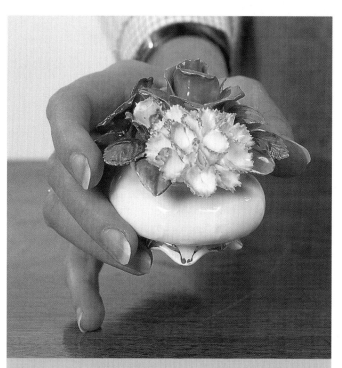

Figure 143 The little finger is used to feel the surface on which a delicate object is being placed. With this fine tactile control the object can be put down with considerable delicacy, even without the use of the eyes. Many valuable objects have been broken due to loss of control of the hand through the little finger.

muscles attached to it and the forcibly outstretched thumb (**Figure 144**). The distal edge is about level with the deep transverse arterial arch and the deep branch of the ulnar nerve. Flexor carpi radialis runs through a separate tunnel beneath.

The flexor tendons in the fingers run through fibrous flexor sheaths, thick over the bones and thin over the joints. The proximal band is derived from the superficial transverse metacarpal ligament at the metacarpal heads, at the distal palmar crease, with other bands at the proximal and middle phalanges (**Figure 144**).

The extensor retinaculum consists of five separate fibro-osseous tunnels over the distal 3 cm or so of the radius (**Figure 145**), plus a sling around and beyond the ulna for extensor carpi ulnaris (see page 54).

Synovial sheaths lubricate the tendons as they pass beneath the retinacular systems, and extend as far as is needed for the tendon's range of movement. The descriptions normally given are in the static state, with the hand in full extension, and so vary from this with movement. Thus, the sheaths on the flexor tendons will move proximally in flexion while those on the extensor tendons will move distally.

Under the flexor retinaculum, the combined palmar synovial sheath (bursa) extends from the proximal wrist crease to the proximal palmar crease (**Figure 144**). Flexor carpi radialis and flexor pollicis longus tendons have separate sheaths running through to their insertion. The tendons to the little finger have an extension from the palmar bursa through to their insertion, but the tendons to the other digits have separate sheaths running on from the level of the distal palmar crease (**Figure 144**).

The dorsal sheaths run from some 3–4 cm proximal to the wrist joint and extend about $^1/_3$ of the way along the metacarpals (**Figure 145**).

1 Abductor pollicis longus
2 Extensor pollicis brevis
3 Extensor carpi radialis longus
4 Extensor carpi radialis brevis
5 Extensor pollicis longus
6 Extensor indicis
7 Extensor digitorum communis
8 Extensor digiti minimi
9 Extensor carpi ulnaris in supination
9* Extensor carpi ulnaris in pronation
10 Extensor retinaculum

1 Digital flexor tendons
2 Flexor pollicis longus
3 Flexor retinaculum
4 Palmar synovial bursa
5 Digital synovial sheaths
6 Superficial transverse metacarpal ligament
7 Digital fibrous flexor sheaths

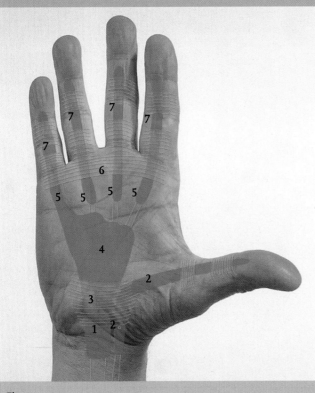

Figure 144

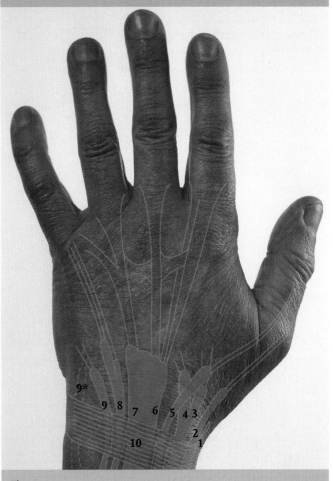

Figure 145

Chapter 6

Vessels and nerves of the arm and hand

THE VESSELS

The main **arterial supply** to the arm comes from the single axillary-to-brachial artery (**Figure 146**), which may make the arm seem vulnerable if this artery is lost. Fortunately, good anastomoses around the shoulder and other joints give adequate protection for the limb under favourable conditions.

From the axilla, the artery runs down in the groove between triceps and coracobrachialis, then biceps, where it can be felt pulsating by pressing against the humerus (see **Figure 88**, page 46), a manoeuvre also controlling arterial bleeding in an emergency. It continues along the medial side of the tendon of biceps, under the bicipital aponeurosis, which separates it from the overlying median cubital vein. Here, about the centre of the upper forearm, it is available for **auscultation when examining blood pressure**.

About level with the neck of the radius it divides into its radial and ulnar branches. The **radial artery** continues over the insertion of biceps. Curving down under brachioradialis, it becomes superficial again to the medial side of its tendon in the lower forearm. Here it lies between the tendons of brachioradialis and flexor carpi radialis on the surface of pronator quadratus and then the radius, where the **radial pulse** is readily palpable (**Figure 147**). Crossing the floor of the 'anatomical snuff-box', under extensor pollicis longus, it winds around the thumb base, then passes between the two heads of the first

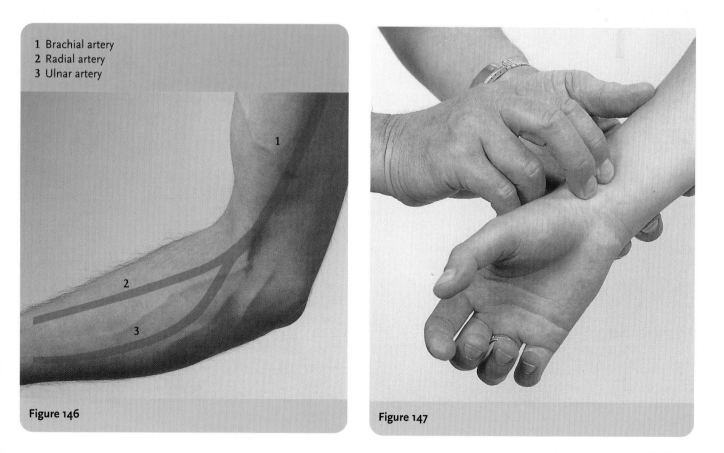

1 Brachial artery
2 Radial artery
3 Ulnar artery

Figure 146

Figure 147

dorsal interosseous and adductor pollicis to enter the deep part of the palm, where it joins with the deep branch of the ulnar artery to form the **deep palmar arch (Figure 148)**.

The **ulnar artery** continues under the superficial flexor muscles, becoming superficial again between the tendons of flexors carpi ulnaris and digitorum superficialis, where its pulse can be felt. The artery then runs with the ulnar nerve, close to the radial side of the pisiform bone, before dividing into superficial and deep branches (**Figure 148**). The **deep branch** crosses the palm with the deep branch of the ulnar nerve to join the radial artery in the deep palmar arch, level with the outstretched thumb and the distal edge of the flexor retinaculum. The **superficial branch** arches across the palm just before the proximal palmar crease, giving branches to each finger via the digital arteries. It is usually described as forming a **superficial palmar arch** with a branch of the radial artery, but the full arch occurs in only 36% of cases, making

the **ulnar artery the main supply to the hand**. Anastomosis occurs between the superficial and deep systems, but this is variable and unreliable. If it is good, the radial artery may play a major role in supplying the hand.

Allen's test gives a quick clinical indication of the relative values in supply. The fingers are compressed firmly into the palm to drive the blood out of the superficial tissues. Firm pressure is then exerted on each artery in turn at the wrist to stop blood flow (**Figure 149A**). On opening the palm, rapid flushing occurs if the free artery is a major supply, but the palm remains white if the compressed artery is of prime importance (**Figure 149B**).

Generally, the ulnar artery is the main supply. Where the radial artery is of subsidiary importance, it and its supported tissues in the forearm, including sections of the radius, can be taken as free grafts, using microsurgical techniques, to replace tissue deficiencies elsewhere in the body.

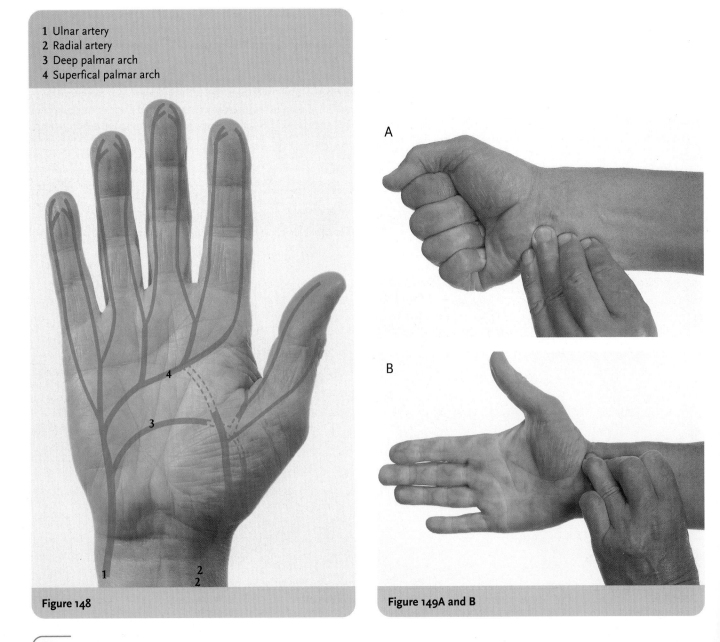

1 Ulnar artery
2 Radial artery
3 Deep palmar arch
4 Superfical palmar arch

Figure 148

A

B

Figure 149A and B

Venous drainage differs from the arterial routes because, although small venae commitantes follow the peripheral arteries, the major veins run superficially and are often visible: these are accompanied by the major lymphatics. Peripherally, the veins are very variable: forming dorsally on each finger, they run in the gutter between the metatarsal heads onto the dorsum of the hand, where—although variable (**Figure 150**)—they often join a dorsal venous arch, whose limbs run to each side of the forearm as the cephalic and basilic veins. The **cephalic vein** follows the radial side (i.e. the cephalic or head side of the limb), crosses the 'anatomical snuff-box', to run up to the cubital fossa (**Figure 151**). Here, a **median cubital vein** links it with the basilic (**Figure 152**). It continues up the arm, over the lateral side of biceps, to reach the deltopectoral groove, before piercing the clavipectoral fascia of the infraclavicular fossa to enter the axillary vein.

The **basilic vein** usually runs up the ulnar border of the arm, anterior to the medial epicondyle (**Figure 152**), where it is joined by the median cubital vein. It then runs in the medial biciptal groove before running deep to join the venae commitantes along the brachial artery, collectively forming the axillary vein.

Traditionally, the **median cubital vein** has been the one of choice for **venipuncture**, usually being large, easy to find even in a fat person and fairly fixed in position. However, the veins on the back of the hand offer many advantages for anaesthesia and infusions without risk to the brachial artery.

The close relationship between the cephalic vein and the radial artery over the radius allows anastomoses to be developed for **renal dialysis**. However, if the radial artery is found to be a major supply to the hand (see *Allen's test*, page 72), the anastomosis may be made after the branch to the superficial palmar arch has been given off, to avoid compromising the hand's circulation.

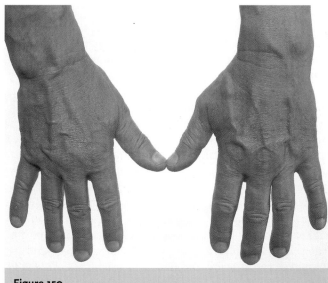

Figure 150

1 Basilic vein
2 Median vein of forearm
3 Cephalic vein
4 Median cubital vein (the median vein in this case joins the median cubital, but more commonly joins the basilic direct)

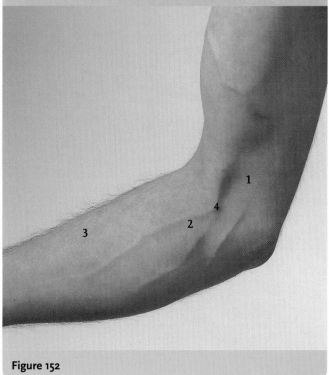

Figure 152

1 Basilic vein
2 Cephalic vein
3 Median cubital vein

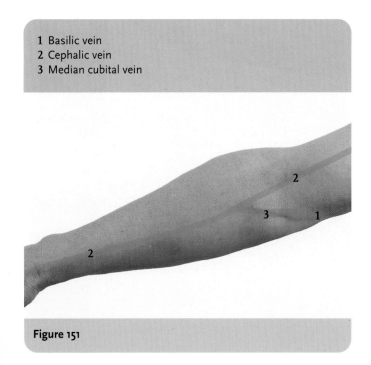

Figure 151

THE NERVES

The upper limb is supplied through the **brachial plexus** with root value C4, C5–C8 and T1. Any neurological examination must consider not only the peripheral nerve of supply but also, on occasions, the roots involved. In the limb the plexus complicates the more simple pattern of segmental supply that is found in the trunk. For the sensory supply, however, the dermatomes of roots remain relatively simple. The area supplied by the central root of the plexus, C7, remains centrally placed, supplying the hand, but cut off more proximally, as are C6 (lateral) and C8 (medial), which supply the forearm; C5 (lateral) and T1 (medial) supply the upper arm. Thus, there is a jump of four segments in the upper arm from lateral to medial, and a jump of two segments in the forearm. The separation zones are narrow, with little overlap, and are known as the **anterior and posterior axial lines**. This is in marked distinction from the very variable overlap (and, to some extent, even area of supply) to be expected between the adjoining segments.

Diagrams of **dermatomes** vary enormously, depending upon their clinical derivation. Hence, it is better to work to a simple pattern and remember that any map can only be an approximation to that found in a particular person.

The nerves supplying areas of skin (**Figure 153**) usually have more than one root, therefore the root value of a particular nerve may seem at variance with the dermatomal map. However, although a nerve may carry neurons from several roots, they do not all supply the whole area supplied by the nerve. Furthermore, although a map of areas of supply may look clear, this is an average picture in which there is enormous variation and, particularly, overlap. For instance, medial or lateral cutaneous nerves of the forearm may be taken as grafts to repair a much more important nerve, such as the median nerve. After removal of the sensory nerve, there may be an area of total sensory loss (rarely approaching that shown on a map),

1 Supraclavicular nerves C3–C4	8* Palmar branch
2 Intercostobrachial T3	8**Posterior branch
3 Upper lateral cutaneous (axillary) C5–C6	9 Median C6–C7
4 Medial cutaneous of arm C8, T1	9* Palmar branch
5 Lower lateral cutaneous (radial) C5–C6	10 Superficial radial C6–C8
6 Medial cutaneous of forearm C8, T1	11 Posterior cutaneous of arm (radial) C6–C8
7 Lateral cutaneous of forearm C5–C6	12 Posterior cutaneous of forearm (radial) C5–C8
8 Ulnar C7–C8	NB The root values given are those of the skin supply.

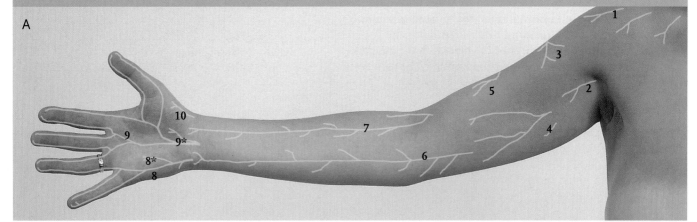

Figure 153A and B

whereas after removal of others, most of the skin retains some protective sensibility because of overlap from adjoining nerves.

The **medial and lateral cutaneous nerves of the forearm** are used on occasions as grafts, hence it is useful to be able to find these easily. The **medial** nerve is a direct branch from the medial cord of the brachial plexus and runs down the arm between biceps and triceps, along with the ulnar nerve to the medial side of the brachial artery. It usually becomes superficial by passing through the same fascial opening through which the basilic vein runs deep [**Figure 153A(6)**]. The vein may be seen in a slim person. The **lateral** nerve, a continuation of the musculocutaneous nerve, runs from between biceps and brachialis, to become superficial about $^2/_3$ of the way down the arm [**Figure 153A(7)**], crossing deep to the median cubital vein close to its junction with the cephalic vein.

Whereas the sensory dermatomes remain relatively simple, the **motor supply** is more complicated. Most muscles receive innervation from more than one root. In the arm, the proximal muscles are innervated by the upper roots of the brachial plexus, with the lower roots running distally. Thus, deltoid receives from C5–C6, whereas the small muscles of the hand are innervated by T1, with some contribution from C8.

The nerves from the brachial plexus have been considered with their muscles of supply (Chapters 4 and 5). The **axillary nerve** (C5–C6), supplying deltoid and teres minor, runs from the posterior cord of the brachial plexus behind the neck of the humerus, some four fingers' breadths below the acromion. Here it is vulnerable to fractures of the neck of the humerus or dislocations of the shoulder joint. The **safe test** for the nerve after an injury is to examine the sensation of the skin over the lower part of deltoid (**Figure 154**).

The **musculocutaneous nerve** (C5–C7) leaves the lateral cord of the brachial plexus, usually in the axilla, passes through coracobrachialis and then between biceps and brachialis (all of which it supplies), before continuing as the lateral cutaneous nerve of the forearm. Loss of the nerve will mean loss of all three muscles, two of which are powerful elbow flexors. Loss of cutaneous supply may only be obvious from a narrow strip along the radial border of the forearm through to the radial styloid (it may replace the radial nerve over the thumb metacarpal).

The **radial nerve** [C5,C6–C8 and T1] is the continuation of the posterior cord of the brachial plexus. It winds around, behind the humerus, in the spiral groove, where, being close to the bone, it is vulnerable in fractures of the middle of the shaft of the bone. If the nerve is cut at this site, the branches supplying triceps and anconeus should be safe because they come off above this level. However, brachioradialis, as well as all the extensors of the wrist and long extensors of the fingers, will lose their innervation, with dropping of the wrist when the hand is held in pronation. The **posterior cutaneous nerve of the forearm** is given off the radial nerve before it enters the groove in about half of cases and when it is in the groove in the others, so its loss will depend upon its origin.

The radial nerve enters the anterior compartment of the arm about $^1/_3$ of the distance above the elbow, coming to lie between brachialis and brachioradialis (**Figure 155**), before running deep to brachioradialis and extensor carpi radialis longus (both of which its supplies), then dividing into its two main branches.

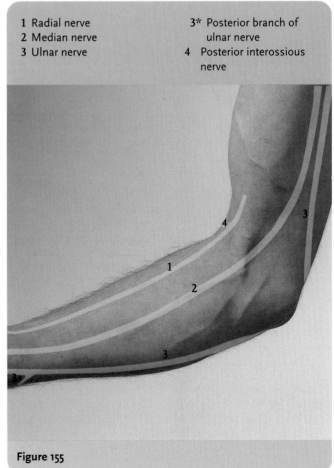

1 Radial nerve	3* Posterior branch of ulnar nerve
2 Median nerve	
3 Ulnar nerve	4 Posterior interossious nerve

Figure 155

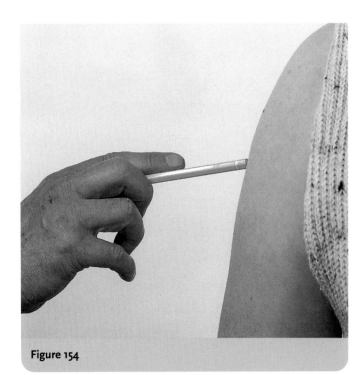

Figure 154

The **posterior interosseous nerve** carries all the motor fibres from the radial nerve and runs through supinator (which it supplies) and around the radius to supply the remaining extensor muscles (**Figure 156**). In 60% of cases the nerve lies on the radius after leaving supinator, where it may be vulnerable to fracture of the bone. If so there will be wrist drop, as in the more proximal radial nerve lesion, but brachioradialis and extensor carpi radialis will be spared.

The **superficial radial nerve** is purely sensory and continues distally under cover of brachioradialis before winding onto the back of the radius, where it may be damaged in fractures. It then runs over the tendons of abductor pollicis longus and extensor pollicis brevis (where, again, it may be damaged or caught up in scars) to supply the back of the hand (**Figure 153(10)**). However, owing to overlap in innervation, loss may be limited to an area over the first dorsal interosseous muscle.

The **ulnar nerve** (C8 and T1 from the medial cord of the brachial plexus plus C7—by a connection from the lateral cord—for flexor carpi ulnaris) runs down the arm fairly superficially (**Figure 155**) and is therefore vulnerable to external injury and compression. It lies initially between coracobrachialis and triceps and then medial to biceps, before going backwards through the intermuscular septum to lie on the medial head of triceps, from where it runs behind the medial epicondyle of the humerus (**Figure 157**). Here it lies in the cubital tunnel created by the bone and the overlying fibres of flexor carpi ulnaris, where it can be damaged by fractures of the bone, direct injury against the bone ('funny-bone') or compression from the overlying fibrous arch of flexor carpi ulnaris (**cubital tunnel syndrome**). Occasionally these overlying fibres are deficient, allowing the nerve to flick around the prominent epicondyle, which can produce the same unpleasant sensation as hitting the 'funny-bone', but here only on movement of the elbow. Just above the elbow it is accessible for anaesthetic nerve block or electrical stimulation.

The ulnar nerve then runs deep to flexor carpi ulnaris and on the surface of the ulnar part of flexor digitorum profundus, both of which it supplies in the upper quarter of the forearm. About 5–7 cm above the ulnar styloid it gives a **dorsal branch**, which carries sensory supply to the backs of the ulnar $1\frac{1}{2}$ digits, as far as the distal interphalangeal joints. The main nerve then runs on, to the radial side of the tendon of flexor carpi ulnaris (**Figure 158**), superficial to the flexor retinaculum and tucked in to the radial side of the pisiform bone, though covered by a fibrous arch and—most importantly—palmaris brevis, which protects it from external pressure, particularly in a power grip (see page 63). Just beyond the pisiform it divides into superficial and deep branches (**Figure 159**). The **superficial branch** supplies palmaris brevis and provides an important sensory supply to the ulnar border of the little finger, and another to the adjoining sides of it and the ring finger, including the nail area.

The **deep branch** passes the hook of the hamate (where it can be compressed) to supply the hypothenar muscles, the interossei, the ulnar two lumbricals, adductor pollicis brevis and, often, the deep head of flexor pollicis brevis.

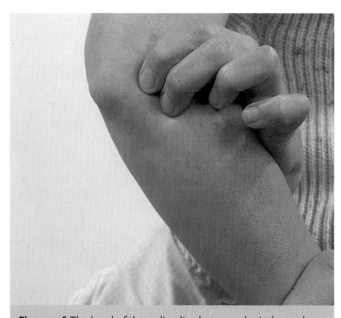

Figure 156 The head of the radius lies between the index and middle fingers. If the other two fingers were placed alongside, the little finger would overlie the posterior interosseous nerve. This is also an excellent site for electrical stimulation of the nerve.

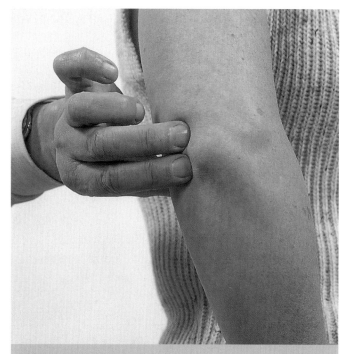

Figure 157 At the elbow the ulnar nerve can often be palpated as it lies above and in the cubital tunnel.

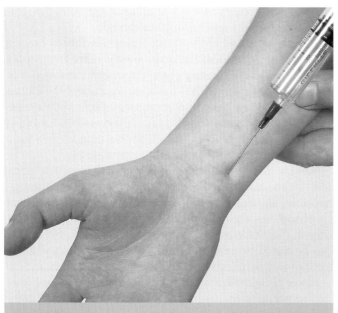

Figure 158 The ulnar nerve is available for local anaestheia or electrical stimulation above the medial epicondyle of the humerous (Figure 157) or as here at the wrist.

1 Ulnar nerve
2 Median nerve
3 Palmar branch of median nerve
4 Deep branch of ulnar nerve
5 Superficial branch of ulnar nerve
6 Thenar branch of median nerve

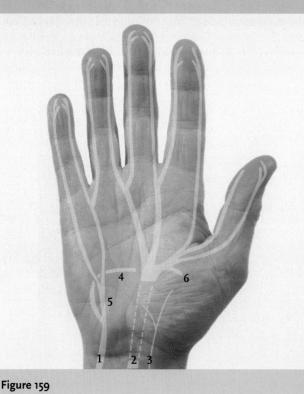

Figure 159

Loss of the ulnar nerve can readily be tested by examination of its sensory area of supply in the hand, which, unlike those of other sensory nerves in the arm, has a fairly sharp cut-off from the median nerve area. The characteristic appearance of ulnar nerve palsy is clawing of the ring and little fingers and sometimes, to a smaller extent, the index and middle fingers (**Figure 160**). This is due to a total loss of the intrinsic muscles of the ulnar two fingers, whereas the lumbricals remain to balance the long muscles of the other two fingers and give interphalangeal extension. If the hyperextension of the metacarpophalangeal joints of the the clawed fingers is prevented, the long extensors can then extend the interphalangeal joints.

Tests for the ulnar nerve can be directed to the individual muscles supplied, but the most usual is to test the interossei (see pages 68 and 69). However, a good simple test for both ulnar and median nerves is to check firm opposition of thumb to little finger. It should be appreciated that loss of the ulnar nerve makes the important oblique power grip impossible, the obliquity of action being entirely due to ulnar-innervated muscle.

The **median nerve** (C5–C8 and T1) is the termination of the lateral and medial cords of the brachial plexus, joined in front of the brachial artery. The nerve runs down the arm with the artery (**Figure 155**), medial to coracobrachialis and then biceps, to the elbow. There it passes under the bicipital aponeurosis, then the arches of the heads of pronator teres and flexor digitorum superficialis (both possible compression sites), supplying both muscles. The nerve is vulnerable to injury and is available for electrical stimulation in the upper arm, medial to biceps, or in the cubital fossa before it runs deep.

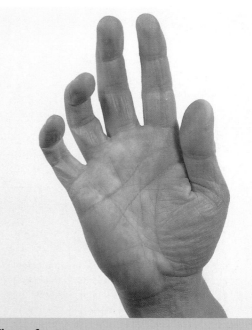

Figure 160

In the forearm the median nerve gives off the **anterior interosseous nerve**, some 2–3 cm distal to the medial epicondyle, to supply flexor pollicis longus, flexor digitorum profundus (to the index and middle fingers) and pronator quadratus. The **main nerve** supplies palmaris longus and flexor carpi radialis and, at the wrist, comes to lie between their tendons, where it is readily available for local anaesthetic block or electrical stimulation (**Figure 161**). The nerve then runs under the **flexor retinaculum** in the line of the proximal part of the thenar crease (**Figure 159**). Here it often becomes compressed (**carpal tunnel syndrome**), usually due to thickening of the synovium of the accompanying tendons (see page 70).

A clinically important small **palmar branch** leaves the main nerve about 5–6 cm above the wrist and, following the line of the flexor carpi radialis, runs superficially over the heel of the hand into the palm. Here it is vulnerable and often cut: although the sensory loss is insignificant, the pain, if a neuroma forms at this point, can be intolerable.

Towards the end of the carpal tunnel the thenar branch leaves to supply the thenar muscles, and the nerve then divides into four terminal sensory branches; one to the radial side of the thumb and one each to the adjoining sides of the thumb and index, the index and middle, and the middle and ring fingers, including the nail-bearing area. The branch to the radial side of the thumb crosses in the region where surgery for a trigger thumb makes it extremely vulnerable.

Loss of the median nerve is the most severe of any in the arm, for the nerve supplies two wrist flexors, the main digital flexors and opposition of the thumb, and is the main sensory supply for the main precision-acting and sensory digits. Loss of the whole median nerve is obvious, but partial loss can be tested by examining for reduced sensibility in the median-innervated area of the hand and reduction in or loss of power of abduction in the thumb (see page 68). These tests can be particularly useful in possible carpal tunnel compression, but electrodiagnostic techniques are more reliable, particularly in the early onset of paraesthesiae in the median nerve sensory area.

Injections in the arm are often required and these must avoid nerves. One site commonly used is into the deltoid muscle, where major nerves can be avoided (**Figure 162**).

Injections of steroids are commonly given to reduce inflammatory activity in cases of carpal tunnel compression. Here it is important to avoid both the ulnar and median nerves and also not to inject the material into tendons. The injection can be given in the region of flexor digitorum superficialis, not more than 1 cm to the ulnar side of palmaris longus, if present. Here it will be between the two nerves and the injecting needle can be eased forwards towards the tunnel, deep to the median nerve, so that the injected material can have maximal effect on the synovial membranes (having first checked on freedom of tendon movement) (**Figure 163**).

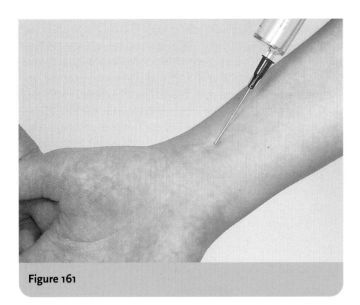

Figure 161

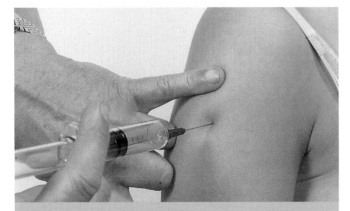

Figure 162 The axillary nerve runs four fingers' breadth below the acromion, but only its terminal branches reach the lateral side, while the radial nerve comes to the lateral side two-thirds of the way to the elbow. These sites are marked by the fingers and so the injection can be safely given into deltoid as shown.

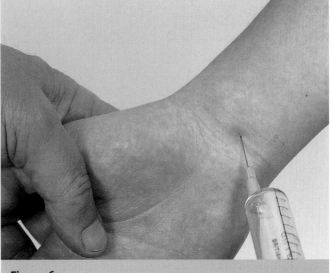

Figure 163

Chapter 7

The back

The axial skeleton has fairly superficial vertebral spines, but the only vertebral bodies lying in a relatively axial position are in the cervical and lumbar regions. The body of L3 is about at the centre of the trunk in a reasonably slim person. The vertebrae are set dorsally in the thorax to allow space for the heart and lungs, also in the sacral region for the birth canal of the female. Hence the column shows its curves—**kyphoses** in the thoracic and sacral regions and **lordoses** in the cervical and lumbar—as obvious features in the back.

Lateral curves may be seen; sometimes to a very mild degree, due to muscular dominance of one side over the other or secondary to poor posture, which, if maintained over a long period, can become fixed. A true **scoliosis** is, however, quite common; it is usually congenital and includes a twist. It can be tested by asking the person to bend forwards, when one side of the back rises above the other.

Of the seven **cervical vertebrae**, C2 (the axis) has a large palpable spine, but those lower are shorter and covered by the ligamentum nuchae. The next prominent one is the so-called vertebra prominens, C7, but the first thoracic is even more prominent.

The **thoracic vertebrae** have long spines that point downwards so that each spine is level with the body of the vertebra below. The eleventh and twelfth become heavier and point more directly backwards, as do the five lumbar spines.

In upright posture, most vertebral spines are not obvious, being sunk between erector spinae muscles in the cervical and lumbar regions, though more prominent in the thoracic and sacral regions.

Because the thoracic spines point downwards and are covered by the supraspinous ligaments and fairly thick skin, they are not easy to examine individually. If, however, the person bends forwards, the spines project much more and can be counted down from C7 and T1 (**Figure 164**). Alternatively, as a line joining the iliac crests crosses the spine of L4, then counting can go upwards from there.

LUMBAR PUNCTURE

The spinal cord only reaches to the lower border of L1, and even in a newborn child to L3, whereas the subarachnoid space extends to about S2. Taking the spine of L4, a needle can be passed into the space below with relative safety. The patient must have the spine fully flexed to open up the intervertebral space, either lying on their side or sitting (**Figure 165**).

The **scapulae** overlie the posterior chest wall, covering the upper seven ribs. The **spine of the scapula** should be readily palpable level with T3 spine (body of T4), and the **inferior angle** level with T8 spine (T9 body). Below the scapula the ribs should be palpable, but close to the vertebrae they are covered by the thick erector spinae muscles. Hence, the twelfth rib, if short, may be impalpable.

The fifth lumbar vertebra and sacrum lie rather deep, the posterior part of the ilium projecting behind the sacrum on

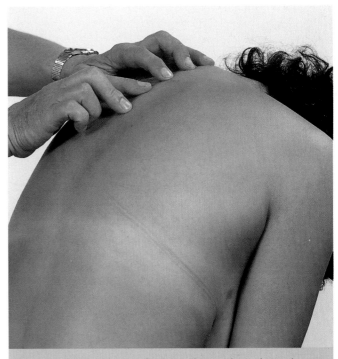

Figure 164 The examining finger can be run down the neck to the vertebra prominens, thence to T1, from where it is possible to count down to L4.

each side. The **posterior iliac spines** are usually easily found, even in an obese person, being overlaid by a dimple in the skin (**Figure 166**).

The **tip of the coccyx** will be found in the upper part of the natal cleft. Above the coccyx the **sacral hiatus** should be at the upper margin of the natal cleft. If the finger is moved up from the coccyx, the depression of the hiatus can be felt in a person who is slim, but less easily in a fat person. It is important to find the hiatus for **caudal or sacral anaesthesia**, where the needle is passed up through the hiatus into the extradural space below the spinal cord (**Figure 167**). The hiatus lies between the two sacral cornua where the neural arch is deficient over the fifth sacral piece. (It may extend higher in spina bifida.) As the dural space ends about S2, anaesthetic injected into the extradural space via the hiatus will anaesthetise the sacral and coccygeal nerves after they have left the dural sac.

Although extradural caudal anaesthesia is preferable and easier, occasionally **block of the individual sacral nerves** is carried out. The posterior superior iliac spine is level with the second sacral spine. The first sacral foramen is about 3 cm above the midpoint between these two spines; the second foramen, the same distance below (**Figure 168**). The lower foramina are on a line sloping inwards from this, with the fourth being level with the sacral cornua (i.e. lateral to the hiatus).

MOVEMENTS OF THE BACK

Movements of the trunk are limited by the basic need for strength, not only for carriage of the upper parts of the body, which may include heavy loads, but also to have a firm base upon which the legs can work.

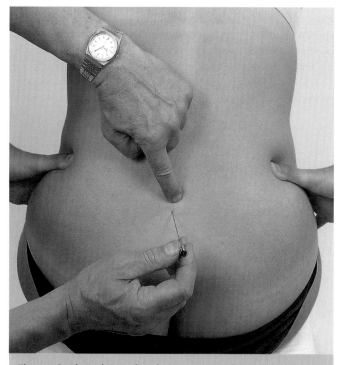

Figure 165 The subject's hands are pressing down above the iliac crests to identify them and, from a line drawn across, the spine of L4 has been marked, the examiner's finger resting on its lower edge. The needle can be passed either above or below the spine (below in this case). After local anaesthetising of the skin, the needle goes in the midline at right angles to the surface, through the supraspinous and interspinous ligaments and the ligamentum flavum and dura, when a release of resistance indicates entry of the space. If the stylus is withdrawn from the needle, a clear fluid should drip out (if normal), confirming the tip is within the space.

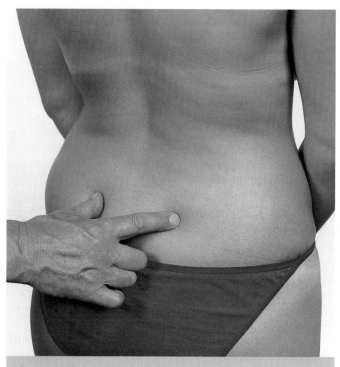

Figure 166 The examiner's index finger and thumb identify the dimples over the posterior superior iliac spine.

Movement in the **upper thoracic spine** is largely directed to respiration and to forming a firm base upon which the arms can operate. It offers some extension, flexion and lateral flexion, but this is limited in extent by the rib cage and sternum. In the **lower thoracic region**, the more flexibly arranged costal cartilages and joints, together with the lower free 'floating ribs', allow greater freedom and, most importantly, offer the **only rotation in the trunk** below the neck. It is this mobility that is so important for the basic positioning of the arms. As the trunk is turned, an S-bend can be seen to have developed in the vertebral column in this region (**Figure 169**).

The **lumbar region** allows for some lateral flexion and a variable amount of flexion and extension from its basic lordotic curve, which even in full flexion is rarely more than straightened, as when touching the toes. The lowest lumbar and lumbosacral region not only takes the greatest load but is also the most vulnerable, with L5 carried, through a thick disc, on the sacrum at a slope of some 45°. It is important to be aware that, other than lateral flexion, all the spinal musculature in the lumbar region is directed towards extension, i.e. increasing the lumbar lordosis and pelvic tilt. Its balancing control comes from the abdominal wall, failure of which is a primary cause of the enormous amount of low-back pathology in the community.

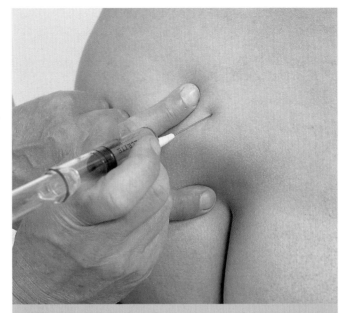

Figure 168 The two fingers mark the posterior superior iliac spine and the sacral cornua, with the needle directed to S2 foramen.

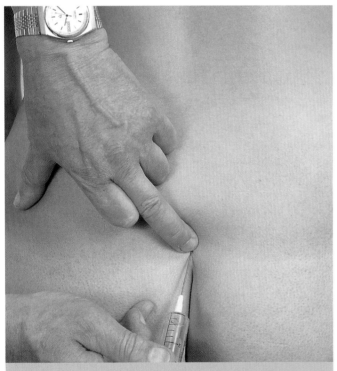

Figure 167 The finger has identified the hiatus and the anaesthetic needle is pointed upwards and forwards at about 45°.

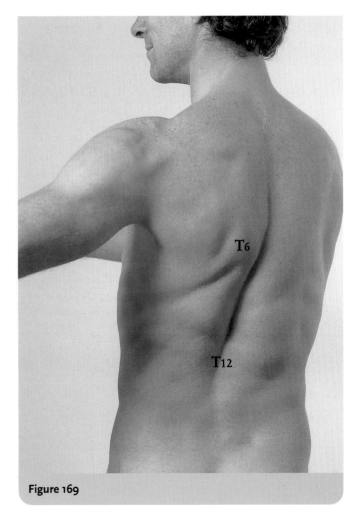

T6

T12

Figure 169

Chapter 8

The thorax, the thoracic wall

The bony skeleton of the thorax is made up of the twelve ribs around each side; linked to the thoracic vertebrae at the back and, the upper ones, to the sternum at the front, through the costal cartilages. The thorax is narrow superiorly, widening below, but the narrowness is masked by the shoulder girdle and its controlling muscles.

Anteriorly, the clavicle overlies the short, flattened but highly curved **first rib, making it normally impalpable**. Its costal cartilage links it directly to the upper and outer angle of the manubrium sterni just below the sternoclavicular joint. If the shoulder is raised, the rib may become palpable just below the medial $^1/_3$ of the clavicle.

The **sternum** has two bony components, the upper broader manubrium and the longer narrower body below, with the short xiphisternal cartilage at the divergence of the costal cartilages. The upper edge of the **manubrium** forms the lower border of the suprasternal notch of the neck. It has a secondary cartilaginous joint with the body of the sternum, which can be felt as a low ridge, about 4 cm below. The manubrium slopes a little, compared with the more vertical sternum below, giving the joint a slight, palpable angulation: the **sternal angle (of Louis) (Figure 170)**. The second costal cartilage articulates with both bones at the sternal angle by synovial joints. As the

ribs run downwards, in passing round the chest wall, the sternal angle is level with the lower border of the fourth thoracic vertebra (4–5 intervertebral disc), i.e. the posterior attachment of the head of the fifth rib.

The ribs articulate with the bodies and transverse processes of the vertebrae of the same number, while the third to the ninth also link with the lower part of the vertebral body above and the intervertebral disc. Anteriorly, the upper seven ribs articulate directly, through their costal cartilages, with the sternum. The eigth, ninth and tenth costal cartilages each turn upwards to articulate with the one above, thus forming the inverted 'V' of the costal margin anteriorly, which, being cartilaginous, has considerable flexibility. The tenth costal cartilage forms the lowest part of the costal margin laterally. The eleventh and the shorter twelfth, so-called floating ribs, are free anteriorly and do not join the costal margin.

Counting the ribs anteriorly is quite easy in a slim male, but may be far less so in a female, owing to the overlying breast. As the first rib lies beneath the clavicle, the **second is the uppermost one which is palpable**. If the examiner's fingers are laid along the ribs, they can be placed in the intercostal grooves, starting with 1–2, with the ribs between them, and then counted down (**Figure 171**).

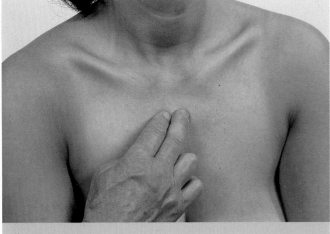

Figure 170

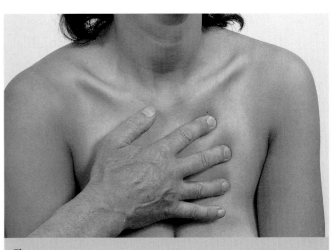

Figure 171

The lower border of the **fifth rib is level with the xiphisternal joint**, while the **linea semilunaris of the abdomen (lateral border of the rectus abdominis muscle) points to the tip of the ninth costal cartilage** (see page 101).

The **levels of the ribs and sternum** are given relative to the vertebrae when at rest: they rise by as much as a vertebra on full inspiration. The shape of the chest is also significant; broad-chested individuals have more horizontally running ribs than slim people. On average, the upper border of the manubrium is level with the body of T3 (a little above its spine), and the lower border (sternal angle) level with T4–T5 (above T4 spine). Lower levels are:

Xiphisternal joint—body of T11 (T10 spine).
Tip of ninth costal cartilage—lower border of L1.
Costal margin (tenth costal cartilage)—L3.

THE BREAST

The breast is often a very prominent feature of an adult female, but in males and prepubertal members of both sexes it is shown only as a small nipple and the surrounding areola. The position of the nipple varies, even in a male, usually being about **1 cm or so outside the midclavicular line** (i.e. a line drawn vertically down from the middle of the clavicle) and lying over the **fourth intercostal space**.

Before puberty the nipple is small and surrounded, in pale-skinned individuals, by a pink areola (**Figure 172**), but is more pigmented if the skin is darker. In males the nipple and areola may become a little more pigmented at puberty, and the nipple more prominent, particularly under cold conditions (**Figure 173**).

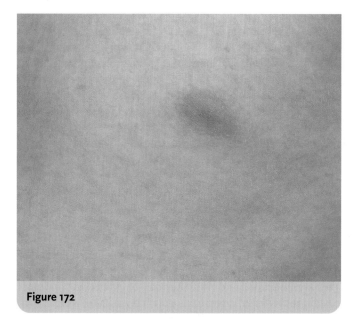

Figure 172

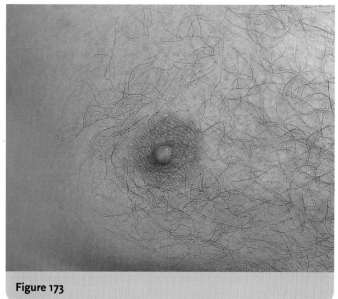

Figure 173

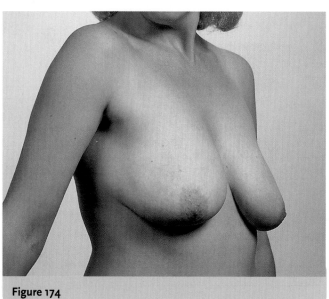

Figure 174

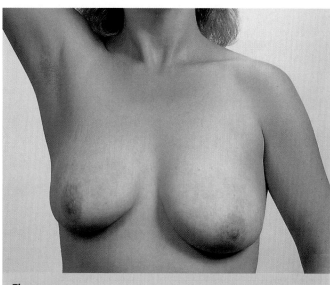

Figure 175

In **females**, around puberty there is a gradual swelling—initially in the region of the nipple—which extends to produce a breast of a size and form characteristic to the individual. The area of the **areola** increases as does the **nipple**, to become obvious features at the apex of the mammary swelling (**Figure 174**). Although very variable in form and size, the breast is essentially a rounded mound, extending **vertically from the second to the sixth ribs; medially from the edge of the sternum to the mid-axillary line**. In this position, some ²/₃ of it overlies the pectoralis major muscle, while the infralateral aspect covers serratus anterior. An important feature is a projection extending along the pectoral muscle towards the axilla: the **axillary tail**. This follows the course of the major lymph-drainage of the breast via the pectoral nodes to the axilla (**Figure 174**). Medially,

the skin remains closely related to the underlying sternum, producing a cleavage between the two breasts.

The breasts are constructed mainly of fatty tissue and lactatory glands. Except for the nipple, the breasts are not directly controlled by muscle. However, **fibrous intersections** within the breast are linked with the fascia over the pectoral muscles and with the skin. Movements of the arms thus affect the breast, not only from the pulling of the skin but also in relation to the pectoral muscle movement, so that raising the arms also pulls up the breast (**Figure 175**). The fibrous connections are particularly strong in the upper part of the gland, where support is most needed. Here they are called the **suspensory ligaments** (of Astley Cooper). They usually give good support in a young and, particularly, nulliparous person, but may become stretched if the breasts are unduly heavy or after multiple pregnancies and lactations.

The role of the suspensory ligaments in maintaining breast-form in the upright posture is evident when the person lies on her back or bends forwards; then the ligaments are less effective in control (**Figures 176A and 176B**). The fibrous intersections in the breast tissue may often become valuable in the **early diagnosis of breast cancer**, when the growth may involve the fibrous tissue, so producing a dimple in the skin, even before a swelling can be palpated. The dimple may become more obvious or only appear when the underlying muscle is put into activity, a fact utilised in procedures advocated for self-examination in women, viewing herself in a mirror.

Pregnancy and lactation lead to hypertrophy and, although the breast may approach normality afterwards, sometimes stretch marks may be left in the skin (**Figure 177**), a feature that may also be seen on the abdomen after pregnancy or in a fat person who slims drastically.

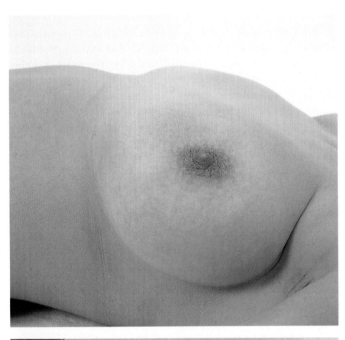

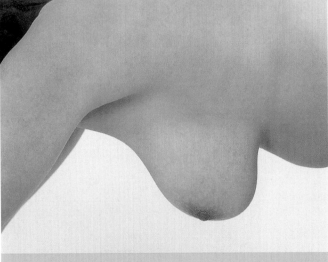

Figure 176A and B The breast illustrated in **figure 175** when lying **(A)** and whenbending forwards **(B)**.

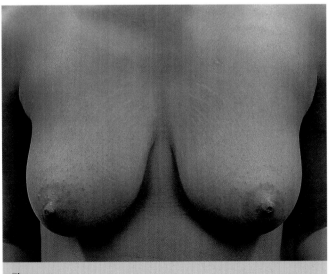

Figure 177

The **nipple and areola** commonly become more pigmented after the first pregnancy; with darker skins, the pigmentation is much greater (**Figure 177**).

The region of the nipple is supplied with **involuntary muscle**, which contracts on stimulation, constricting the areola and erecting the nipple (**Figures 178A and B**), a feature that increases during lactation, when the nipple hypertrophies for suckling.

Small swellings are apparent in the areola (**Figure 178A**), caused by the **areolar glands**. These are specialised sebaceous glands that enlarge during pregnancy, producing an oily secretion to assist in lubricating the skin of the nipple during lactation, thus maintaining it in a supple healthy state.

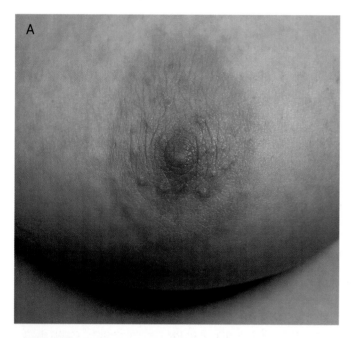

Figure 178A and B The effect of cold on the nipple is readily seen in **B** as compared with **A**.

BLOOD SUPPLY OF THE BREAST

The breast receives its main blood supply from three sources: perforating branches from the internal thoracic artery, medially [**Figure 179(left 1)**]; lateral thoracic branches from the axillary artery, laterally (**2**); and the acromiothoracic artery (**3**), with venous drainage following the same routes. The vessels form a rich **subareolar plexus**, while the medial and lateral supplies converge and anastomose, mainly below the nipple. Here the veins may be seen through the skin, particularly when enlarged during pregnancy and lactation. Thus, circumferential incisions in the lower part of the breast not only avoid major blood vessels but also follow resting stress lines (see page 2).

Lymphatics of the breast are of major clinical importance as a route for the spread of cancer of the breast. It is often said that drainage tends to follow segmental routes, but such a description can be misleading. By far the most common route is along the pectoralis muscle—mainly its fascia—via pectoral lymph nodes [**Figure 179(right 1)**], thence to central and apical lymph nodes (**2**), from where main drainage is into the venous system of that side of the body. Spread does occur upwards to infra- and supraclavicular lymph nodes (**3**), medially to nodes along the internal thoracic vessels (**4**), and downwards into the upper abdomen and even the inguinal nodes (**5**). Spread to the other breast (**6**) and thence axilla is described, but the less usual routes may only open up when the primary routes are blocked by secondary involvement.

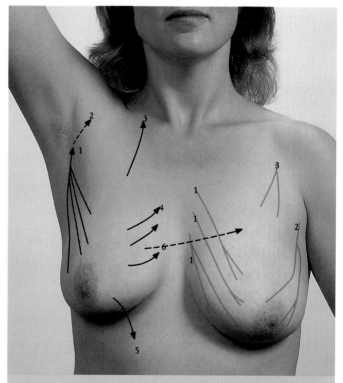

Figure 179 Lymph drainage of the breast shown on the right in black and arterial supply on the left in red. (Figures as in text.)

SURFACE REPRESENTATION ON THE CHEST WALL

The **sternal angle (of Louis)**—the junction of the manubrium and the body of the sternum—is at the level of the lower part of T4 (T4–T5 disc). It is a very important surface level in the thorax because of the number of underlying structures (**Figure 180**).

The **aorta** arches backwards and a little to the left, behind the lower half of the manubrium sterni and thus just above the sternal angle, reaching the lower left aspect of T4 vertebra, and runs down then close to the vertebral bodies. The left **brachiocephalic vein** lies immediately behind the upper half of the manubrium, as it crosses to join the right vein to form the **superior vena cava**, which runs down the right border of the manubrium and sternum. This is joined by the **vena azygos** at the level of the sternal angle, having arched forwards over the **root of the right lung**.

The **trachea** runs down to the sternal angle, dividing to form the main bronchi, which diverge to run to the hila of the lungs. The **upper parts of the hila** are at the level of the angle; here, also, the **pulmonary artery** runs under the arch of the aorta to divide into its branch to each lung. In the fetus the left pulmonary artery is joined to the aorta by the **ductus arteriosus**, but after birth this constricts, due to the reduction in oxygen tension, and—ceasing to carry blood—forms the **ligamentum arteriosum**, around which the **left recurrent laryngeal nerve** turns upwards from the vagus. The **superficial cardiac nerve plexus** lies in front of the ligamentum arteriosum, with the **deep** one behind. These receive parasympathetic contributions from the vagus and sympathetic from the cervical sympathetic trunk.

The **thoracic duct** begins its course upwards in the thorax to the right, but crosses over to the left near T4–T5.

THE PLEURA AND LUNGS

The lungs form the greatest volume of the thoracic contents and, because of their role, this volume varies with the phase and needs of respiration. The **pleura has a parietal layer** that conforms with the movements of the thoracic walls and a **visceral layer** that moves with the lungs. The parietal layer lines the thorax to the maximal extent of inflation of the lungs. Thus, in the resting stages of respiration there is a marked difference in the extent of pleural cover of the thoracic walls and of the lungs within. The main differences are on the costal and diaphragmatic margins, where the potential space of these recesses can be filled by the lungs as the depth of respiration increases. In these **costodiaphragmatic recesses** the two parietal layers of pleura are in contact, but will be separated on expansion of the lungs. Elsewhere the lungs generally conform to the pleural lining of the chest wall (**Figure 181**).

The **lung apex or dome of the thoracic cavity** extends about 2–3 cm above the medial $^1/_3$ of the clavicle in quiet respiration. It is covered by the **suprapleural membrane (Sibson's fascia)**, which extends from the tubercle of the transverse process of

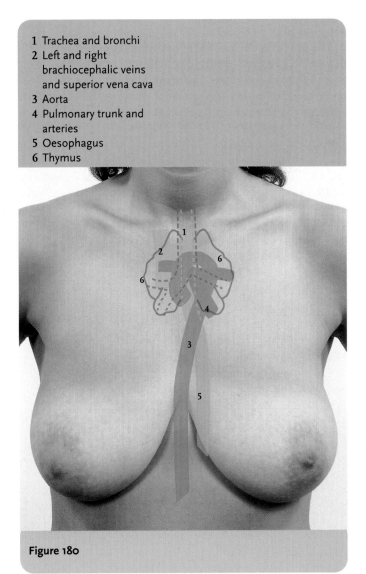

1 Trachea and bronchi
2 Left and right brachiocephalic veins and superior vena cava
3 Aorta
4 Pulmonary trunk and arteries
5 Oesophagus
6 Thymus

Figure 180

C7 vertebra to the inner margin of the first rib, supported in about 50% of cases by muscle, the **scalenus minimus**. In addition, the dome is protected anteriorly and laterally by the scalene muscles

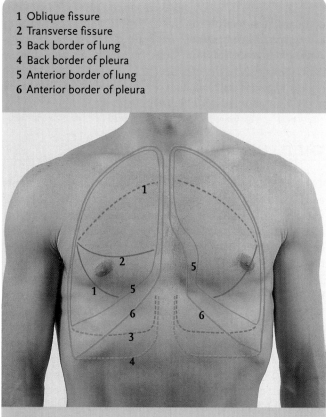

1 Oblique fissure
2 Transverse fissure
3 Back border of lung
4 Back border of pleura
5 Anterior border of lung
6 Anterior border of pleura

Figure 181

and anteriorly by sternomastoid. As part of the projection of the lung above the clavicle is due to the slope of the first rib, in deep inspiration the chest wall will be raised and with it the clavicle, so reducing the height of the dome above it. For a similar reason, the height is greater in asthenic than in broad-chested individuals.

From the medial $^1/_3$ of the clavicle, both pleura and lung follow the chest wall closely except at the sternal margin (and at the lung fissures). The sternal reflection of the **pleura** crosses the sternoclavicular joint to approach the midline at the sternal angle, the two pleurae then running down close together. On the right side the pleura turns laterally at the junction of the seventh costal cartilage and the sternum, and then follows around the chest wall behind the eighth rib at the midclavicular line, the tenth rib at the mid-axillary line and the twelfth rib below the medial border of the scapula (lateral margin of erector spinae). Medial to this it runs below the twelfth rib, towards the transverse process of L1 vertebra, to form a subcostal pleural triangle. Here the pleural cavity is often said to be vulnerable, particularly in surgical exposure of the kidney; however, it is protected by the quadratus lumborum and erector spinae muscles. The danger is when the twelfth rib is very short; the incision can then run up, unintentionally, to the eleventh rib.

On the left side the pleura runs to the fourth costal cartilage, where a cardiac notch takes the pleura out to the left of the sternum, down to the seventh costal cartilage; the lower margin then follows the same course as on the right side. Posteriorly, both lungs and pleurae have a medial margin some 2–3 cm lateral to the midline, i.e. along the vertebral bodies, except on the left side where the aorta intervenes.

Anteriorly, **the lung** follows behind the sternum, with only a slight separation from the pleural reflection on the right, down to the level of the sixth costal cartilage. From

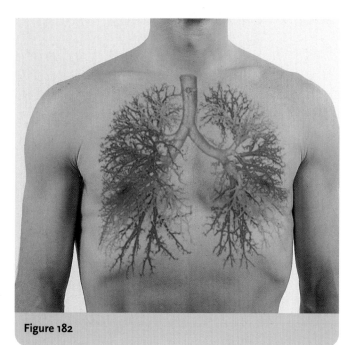

Figure 182

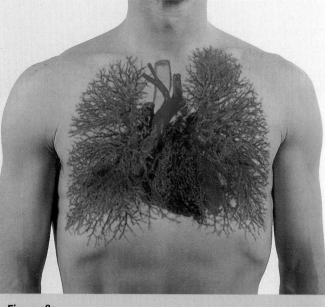

Figure 183

here it follows around the chest wall some two ribs above the pleural reflection, i.e. sixth, eigth and tenth ribs at the three lines. On the left side, the cardiac notch takes the lung laterally by 2–3 cm opposite the fifth costal cartilage and then moving in a little at the sixth, before following the same lower course as on the right (**Figure 181**).

The lines of lung markings relative to the costodiaphragmatic recesses and the cardiac notch are essentially those at rest, but will not vary much in quiet respiration. In deep respiration, however, the lungs will expand towards the limits of the pleural recesses.

LUNG FISSURES

The left lung is divided into two lobes—an upper and a lower—by the oblique fissure. The right lung has an oblique and a transverse fissure dividing it into upper, middle and lower lobes. The oblique fissures of the lungs can be shown on the surface by a line drawn around the chest wall from 2–3 cm from the midline at the back, a little below the spine of T3 vertebra, to the sixth costal cartilage anteriorly. It also follows the medial border of the scapula when the arm is raised above the head. The transverse fissure lies anteriorly behind the fourth costal cartilage and runs horizontally laterally to meet the oblique fissure in the mid-axillary line. The transverse fissure passes above the nipple in the male, while the oblique fissure passes below it, though both run below in deep inspiration.

BRONCHOPULMONARY SEGMENTS

The anatomy of the lung is based on the repeatedly dividing bronchi, the bronchial tree, and—like in a tree—each branch is a self-contained unit (**Figure 182**). Blockage of a bronchial branch removes aeration of that segment, which will collapse as the air is absorbed. The branches of the pulmonary artery run in close parallel with the bronchi and are likewise directed only to that particular segment, as are the veins (**Figure 183**). This bronchopulmonary segmental pattern and the positions of the segments are therefore of major clinical importance (**Figure 184**).

Superior lobe:	Right middle lobe:	5 InferiorLower lobe:	10 Subapical (present in
1 Apical	4 Lateral	6 Lower apical	50% of cases, reducing in
2 Posterior	5 Medial	7 Anterior basal	this case the inferior and
3 Anterior	**Left lingular lobe:**	8 Lateral basal	lateral basal segments)
	4 Superior	9 Posterior basal (medial	
		basal not seen)	

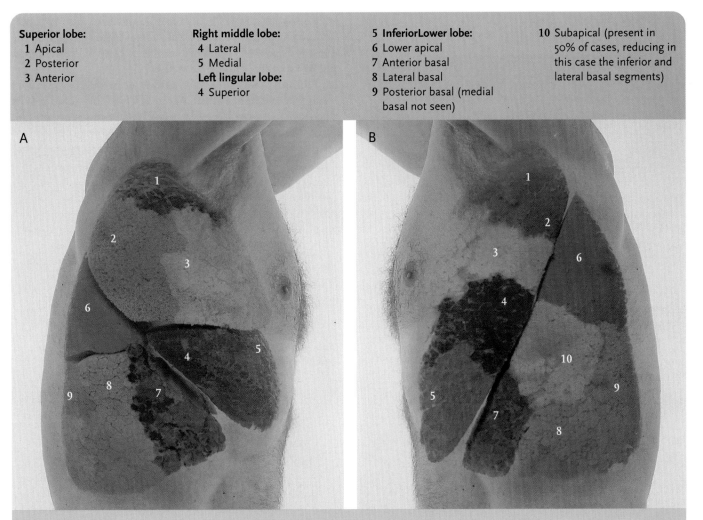

Figure 184A and B

Examination of the lungs initially concerns the effective inspiration and expiration of air, which depends upon the movements of the chest wall. These can be observed quite simply as the patient breathes, but variations between the two sides are less obvious. If the two hands are placed with the fingers to the sides of the chest and the thumbs touching in the midline in expiration, as the patient breathes in, the thumbs will normally be pulled apart to an equal amount on each side.

Being air-filled, the chest **resonates** to the person's voice and also to **percussion**, rather like a drum. The extent of normal lung can be estimated by percussion. The middle finger (usually) is placed palmar surface against the chest wall and hit by the tip of the bent middle finger of the other hand, the movement occurring at the wrist (**Figure 185**). The air-filled region gives a resonant sound, but this beomes dull if there is solid tissue or fluid beneath. By this means it is possible to indicate if there is consolidation in the lung, or fluid in the pleural cavity or fissures. **Auscultation**, as by a stethoscope, allows the observer to hear variation from the normal sounds of airflow during breathing and also qualities of resonance to voice.

THE HEART

The heart fills the central part of the thorax (the **middle mediastinum**) and is covered by a loose fibrous coat (the **fibrous pericardium**), which has a lubricating lining (the **serous pericardium**) to cut friction as the heart beats. From its central position the **apex** extends to the left (**Figure 186**). The heart's shape and position vary, not only due to its own beating but also with respiration. As the diaphragm is lowered during inspiration the heart lies more vertically (appearing narrower in a radiograph), becoming more transverse in expiration. The apex and apex beat therefore vary with the phase of respiration. In a broad-chested individual and those with a naturally higher diaphragm, the heart lies more transversely, whereas a narrower-chested individual will have a more vertical heart. Distension of the stomach can push the heart over to the right, so that overeating can materially embarrass an already stressed and particularly dilated heart. The actual contractile state of the heart also affects its appearance, added to which—owing mainly to the twist of the intermuscular septum—the heart rotates a little to the right on contraction (systole).

All these changes can affect the position of the apex and apex beat, which is usually described as being just inside the midclavicular line in the fifth intercostal space. The apex beat is that part of the heart that can normally be felt against the chest wall; however, as this is usually so close to the true apex, the two tend to be treated together.

From the front, the right border of the heart is made up entirely of the **right atrium** [**Figure 186(1)**]. The **superior vena cava** (**2**) runs down the right side of the manubrium and

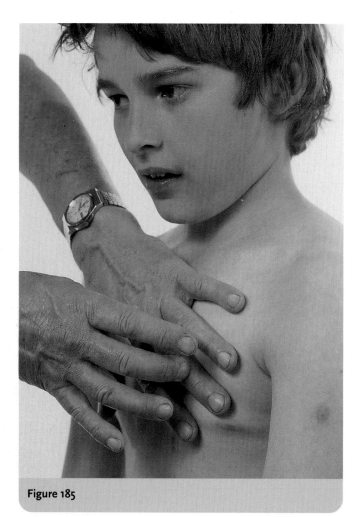

1	Right atrium	5	Pulmonary artery
2	Superior vena cava	6	Left auricle
3	Inferior vena cava	7	Left ventricle
4	Arch of the aorta	8	Right ventricle

Figure 185

Figure 186 (Surface details as also shown in Figure 187.)

sternum, to enter the atrium level with the third costal cartilage. The **atrium** curves a little outside the right border of the sternum to the sixth costal cartilage or the xiphisternal joint. The **inferior vena cava** enters from below (**3**). On the left side the **arch of the aorta** (**4**) lies behind the lower half of the manubrium sterni with the **pulmonary artery** (**5**) just below, forming a bulge with its branch evident on an anteroposterior radiograph. The two arteries form the aortic and pulmonary knuckles of the radiograph. Below this and extending 2.5 cm to the left of the sternum, and behind the second intercostal space and the third costal cartilage, there is a small portion of the **left auricle** (**6**). The rest of the left border of the heart is made up of the **left ventricle** (**7**).

The lower border of the heart has the inferior vena cava opening to the right, with the remainder made up of ²/₃ **right ventricle** (**8**) and the apical ¹/₃ , **left ventricle**, though the latter increases a little in systole owing to the twist of the heart.

As the **left ventricle** runs behind the right, it forms the posterior aspect towards the apex, with the **left atrium** forming the major upper part of the heart. This lies immediately in front of the oesophagus, so that left atrial dilatation tends to compress the oesophagus, producing difficulty in swallowing (dysphagia), a common feature of left-sided problems in the heart.

The **valves of the heart** all lie surrounded by a fibrous ring, on which both atrial and ventricular muscles are mounted. Because of the obliquity of the heart in the chest, the valves lie on a line from the medial end of the third left costal cartilage, downwards and to the right, towards the right border of the sternum, level with the fourth intercostal space. They lie, from left to right, pulmonary (PV), aortic (AV; a little behind the pulmonary), then mitral (MV), a little behind the

tricuspid (TV) (**Figure 187**).

The **transverse pericardial sinus** runs above the heart, between the two great arteries and the veins, and is level with the sternal angle. The **oblique sinus** lies behind the ventricles.

CLINICAL EXAMINATION OF THE HEART

Observation in a slim person may show evidence of pulsation at the apex beat, usually in the fifth intercostal space, particularly if the person is seen after exercise or is bending forwards to bring the heart closer to the chest wall.

Palpation of the apex beat is usually quite easy in a slim male, if the fingers are separated and laid along the intercostal spaces (**Figure 188**). In all but small-breasted females or in a more obese male it is less easy. In a female the hand should be laid beneath the breast (see overleaf, **Figure 189** see overleaf). Difficulty in palpation may be helped if the person leans forwards.

A rough estimation of heart size may be made by **percussion**, using the same technique as for the lungs (**Figure 185**). If the finger is laid on the chest wall, parallel to but outside the heart, percussion will show lung resonance. The finger is then brought nearer until the sound changes to the dullness expected over a solid body. By repeating this process around the heart, a reasonably good clinical map can be produced, though not as accurate as by radiography, ultrasound, etc. It is less effective in a barrel-shaped chest, where overlying lung tissue may blur the edges.

Listening to the sounds generated by blood flow and valve closure etc. (i.e. **auscultation**) can give valuable information even when carried out by a simple stethoscope. It is important to be aware that the sound is propagated via the blood

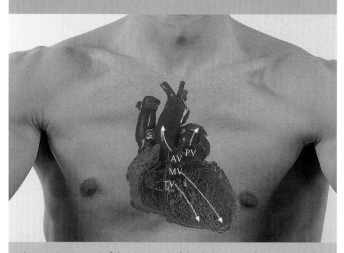

PV = Pulmonary valve
AV = Aortic valve
MV= Mitral valve
TV = Tricuspid valve

The arrows indicate the direction of the blood flow and extend to the sites for auscultation of the valves.

Figure 187 A cast of the cavities of the heart and the origins of the great vessels with the heart in diastole. The coronary arteries can be seen in red, coursing over the surface of the cast of the heart.

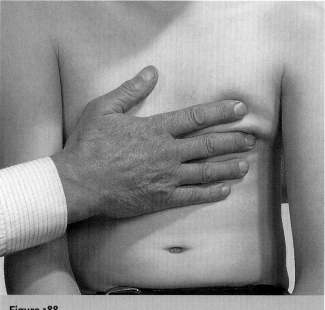

Figure 188

after it has passed a valve. There is little point, therefore, in listening over the valves. The mitral and tricuspid sounds must be looked for below and to the left of the valves, i.e. over the ventricles, while the mitral is best heard over the apex. The aortic and pulmonary sounds can be heard over the origins of these vessels, above the valves (**Figure 187**).

OTHER THORACIC STRUCTURES

The **thymus gland** lies immediately behind the manubrium and sternum, and in an adult it is a lobulated structure extending from the upper border of the manubrium down to the fourth costal cartilages (**Figure 180**, page 87). As it develops from the third branchial pouch and moves down into the thorax, its position is rather variable, though not as much as the inferior parathyroid, which, developing from the same pouch, can be anywhere from behind the thyroid to the thorax with the thymus.

The **aorta** leaves the heart behind the sternum, roughly level with the third costal cartilage and runs upwards, towards the right border before arching backwards and slightly to the left, behind the lower half of the manubrium sterni. It meets the lower part of the body of T4 vertebra, then descends along the bodies of the thoracic vertebrae, producing a slight flattening that gradually moves to the front as the artery leaves the thorax through the diaphragm in front of T12 (i.e. about 7–8 cm below the xiphisternal joint) (**Figure 190**).

The **oesophagus** enters the thorax in the midline behind the trachea (**Figure 180**). The position of the **trachea** can be seen as a band of greater translucency in a radiograph, in the centre of the vertebral bodies, until it divides at the level of the sternal angle. The oesophagus, although pushed slightly to the right by the aorta at T4, carries on downwards in front of the aorta, moving to the left to leave the thorax opposite T10, about 2–3 cm to the left and 4–5 cm below the xiphisternal joint.

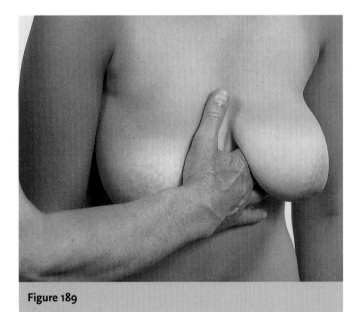

Figure 189

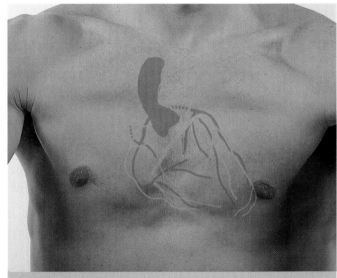

Figure 190 Surface projection of the coronary arteries (red) and veins (blue). The two coronary arteries run from the sinuses above the left and right anteriro aortic valves. The right artery runs around the heart in the atrioventricular groove. The left runs behind the pulmonary artery posteriorly into the atrioventricular groove, having given the very important anterior interventricular artery. The cardiac veins terminate mainly in the coronary sinus which enters the back of the right atrium, though anterior cardiac veins enter separately.

A = Aorta	8	Atrial branch of left coronary
P = Pulmonary artery	9	Coronary sinus
1 Right coronary	10	Great cardiac vein
2 Left coronary	11	Posterior vein of left ventricle
3 Right marginal	12	Anterior cardiac
4 Posterior interventricular	13	Middle cardiac
5 Anterior interventricular		
6 Left marginal		
7 Circumflex branch of left coronary		

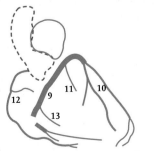

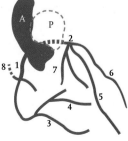

Chapter 9

The abdomen

THE ABDOMINAL WALLS

The diaphragm is a musculotendinous roof to the abdomen, arching upwards into the thorax. It is lower in the middle, where it is tendinous below the heart, than on the two sides; higher on the right, where it overlies the liver (see **Figure 206**, page 103), than on the left, where it overlies the stomach. Anteriorly its fibres are short, with longer fibres around the inside of the lower six costal cartilages and the adjoining ribs. Posteriorly the crura give the main downward pull so that the lowering is far greater on the base of the lungs than on the heart.

The level of the diaphragm depends not only on the state of respiration but also on the person's build, lying relatively higher in a broad-chested individual than in a narrow-chested one. In a neutral respiratory position, the right side of the dome is usually level with the fifth costal cartilage (T10–T11 or fourth rib in the midclavicular line) and the left with the sixth costal cartilage (T11–T12 or fifth rib), with the central portion level with the xiphisternal joint . However, it may be a full vertebra higher, with the left side raised more, dependent upon the contents of the stomach. The diaphragm tends to be higher if the person is supine, and one or other side may be raised when lying on that side. When sitting or in a half lying–sitting position and the abdominal wall most relaxed, the diaphragm sinks to its lowest level. This is why people with respiratory problems (dyspnoea) prefer to sleep half-sitting, finding breathing difficult when the diaphragm is raised when lying flat.

During quiet respiration, the diaphragm moves little more than 1 cm in height. In deep or forced respiration, its vertical range varies between individuals, being anything from 3 to 10 cm.

The **motor and most of the sensory nerve supply** of the diaphragm come, via the **phrenic nerve**, from cervical roots; mainly from C4, with quite large contributions from C5 and smaller ones from C3. The nerve runs down **over scalenus anterior**, where it can be stimulated electrically to induce breathing or be anaesthetised to still the diaphragm, as in persistent hiccup or diaphragmatic pain (see page 31). Although a small peripheral sensory innervation comes from the local intercostal nerves, the major supply is from the phrenic nerve, which explains why pain from the diaphragm may be referred to skin areas supplied by the same cervical roots.

ANTERIOR ABDOMINAL WALL

The anterior abdominal wall is made up of a dynamic 'corset' of three sheets of muscle, each running in a different direction, on each side. These are incorporated by their fibrous aponeuroses into controlling sheaths around the longitudinally running pair of rectus muscles anteriorly, thus giving a close functional interrelationship between all muscle components of the wall, particularly above the umbilicus.

The **rectus abdominis** comes from a broad superior muscular attachment to the 5–7 costal cartilages and runs down to a narrower attachment to the pubic crest. It has three tendinous intersections in the anterior parts of each muscle; one below the xiphisternum, one between this and the umbilicus and $^1/_3$ at the umbilicus. These divisions can be seen quite easily in a reasonably slim male (**Figure 191**). As the fibrous intersections are attached to the anterior wall of the rectus sheath, this arrangement allows for the remarkably fine control possible in the supra-umbilical part of the anterior abdominal wall. **Innervation** is from the **lower six intercostal nerves**.

Externus obliquus abdominis is attached by fleshy slips to the outer aspects of the lower eight ribs. The upper four slips interdigitate with the lower four of serratus anterior and below that with latissimus dorsi. These digitations are readily visible in a slim muscular male (**Figure 192**). The lowest fibres run downwards to the anterior part of the iliac crest. The higher ones run downwards and forwards, forming a tendinous aponeurosis (the change often visible in a curved line from the ninth costal cartilage to the anterior superior iliac spine), to form a major part of the anterior wall of the rectus sheath, meeting its fellow of the other side at the linea alba. The lowest part of the aponeurosis contributes to the inguinal ligament.

Internus obliquus abdominis lies deep to the external oblique, and its upper fibres run at right angles to it, i.e. upwards and medially. The lowest attachment is to the outer $^2/_3$ of the inguinal ligament, above that to the anterior part of the iliac crest and then the thoraco-lumbar fascia. The upper fibres run to the margins of the lower ribs. Below that, the aponeurosis joins the rectus sheath, but at the arcuate line, below the umbilicus, the aponeuroses of all three muscles run only anterior to rectus.

Transversus abdominis forms the deepest layer and is the prime abdominal constrictor (**Figure 193**). The lowest fibres come from the inguinal ligament and join with the internal oblique in controlling the inguinal canal. The rest of the muscle comes from the iliac crest, the thoraco-lumbar fascia and the inner aspect of the lower six ribs, these latter fibres interdigitating with the diaphragm. The fibres run medially, become aponeurotic and run into the posterior wall of the rectus sheath, except below at the arcuate line, where they join the anterior wall.

The three muscles are supplied by the **lower intercostal nerves and L1**.

The functions of the abdominal muscles are more complex than the obvious one of support for the abdominal contents. A degree of compression needs to be maintained to influence venous return to the low-pressure thorax and a periodic increase of pressure is needed for expulsive forces, defecation and urination, as well as vomiting and parturition.

The **rectus abdominis muscles** are the prime flexors of the lumbar spine but can exert no local control, particularly over the vulnerable lower lumbar region. The **oblique muscles** are important rotatory-flexor muscles acting on the lower thoracic vertebrae: the external muscle, on one side, working with the internal and on the other side, through the intervening aponeurosis, giving elegant control of the upper trunk on the lower. The upper musculature, and the **transversus** in particular, can play an important part in fine respiratory control. Full compressor activity of the abdominal muscles on the essentially incompressible abdominal contents is vital in support of the back in heavy lifting. A similar, more local effect should come from the muscles below the umbilicus, where the aponeurosis of all three muscles runs in front of the rectus; by compressing the lower abdominal contents, they, in turn, support the lower lumbar and lumbosacral spine, which is otherwise so vulnerable to injury. A failure of this latter support is the cause of so much low-back disability in the community (**Figure 194**).

The skin and superficial tissues on the anterior abdominal wall show some specialisation. The skin is much thinner and more sensitive than the thicker skin of the back and shows characteristic hair patterns. Below the umbilicus there are increasing amounts of membranous tissue in the superficial fascia, condensing to form the **suspensory ligament of the penis** in

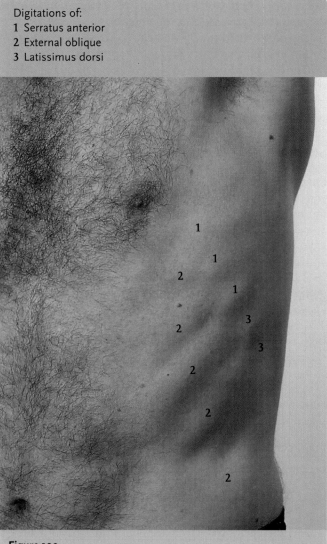

Digitations of:
1 Serratus anterior
2 External oblique
3 Latissimus dorsi

Figure 192

1 Rectus abdominis
2 Tendinous intersections
3 Inguinal ligament
4 External oblique muscle
5 Medial border of external oblique
6 Linea semilunaris
7 Linea alba

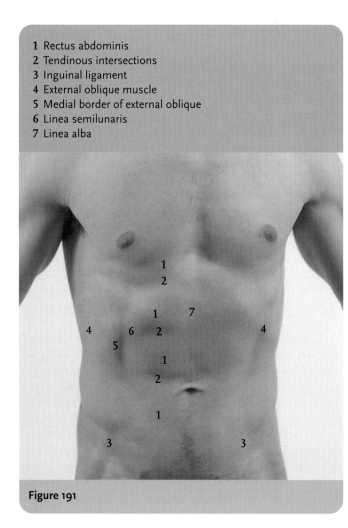

Figure 191

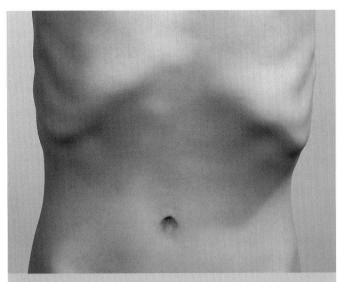

Figure 193 In maximal forced expiration with contraction of the abdominal wall, the constricting effect of the transversus abdominis muscles can be seen, acting from within the rib cage. In order to achieve this degree of abdominal contraction, the other abdominal muscles must relax so that they can be pulled in with the wall. However, their lower fibres remain active in support of the subumbilical region.

males and the **mons pubis** in females. The membranous layer extends into the perineum to be attached to the posterior margin of the **perineal membrane**, behind the genitalia. Any fluid, such as urine from a ruptured urethra, is therefore free to track up into the abdominal wall. As the skin is bound down at the inguinal folds (the flexion creases between abdomen and leg) to the deep fascia of the leg, this prevents any fluid tracking down into the legs.

INGUINAL REGION

This is an important region clinically, particularly in a male, as it includes the passage serving and linking the testis with the abdominal cavity and is hence a potential site for herniation as well as other problems. During embryological and fetal development, a column of mesenchyme, the **gubernaculum testis**, extends from the intra-abdominal testis, maintaining an undifferentiated channel through the developing abdominal wall and a core for the scrotum. Shortly before birth this is invaded by the **processus vaginalis,** which comes from the abdomen and through which the testis descends to the scrotum; the processus vaginalis normally then closes. The **inguinal canal** remains as an oblique canal, running through the muscles of the lower abdominal wall, immediately above and parallel to the inguinal ligament, carrying the ductus deferens and the vessels and nerves of the testis (**Figure 196**).

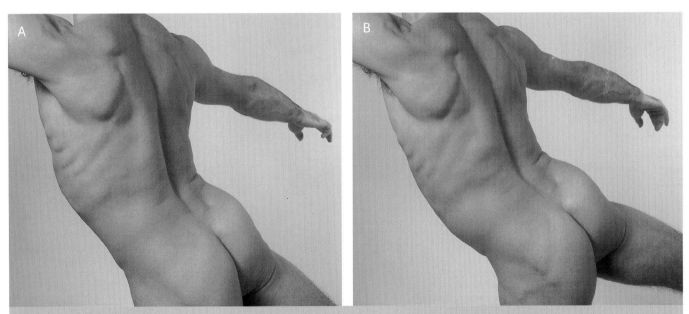

Figure 194A and B It is common for the strength of the back and trunk to be equated with the strength of the back muscles. This is far from the truth. These muscles certainly extend the spine and give the fine control of the vertebrae, but the strength comes from the abdominal muscles, which compact the abdominal contents. In the arabesque of classical ballet, the back needs to be arched to carry the working leg into full extension. Here the abdominal muscles are vital to give strength to the back (**A**). The abdominal muscles have been allowed to relax(**B**). Control of trunk rotation becomes less accurate. Far more important, the smooth curve through the lumbar spine is lost for sharper angulation in the lower lumbar and lumbosacral region, the most vulnerable section of the spine. For this reason, the term 'arabesque back' has been coined to describe the painful lower back common in poorly trained dancers.

The **inguinal ligament** represents the lower border of the aponeurosis of the external oblique muscle of the abdomen, here joined to the deep fascia of the leg. Behind the inguinal ligament another channel links the abdomen with the leg, the **femoral sheath**, containing three passages: medially a fat-supported lymphatic channel, the **femoral canal**; then the **femoral vein and the artery**, with the **femoral nerve** more laterally, outside the sheath (**Figure 195**). Like the inguinal canal, the femoral canal is a possible site for **hernia** and, their positions being close, it is important to be able to differentiate one from the other. An **inguinal hernia** comes from just above the inguinal ligament, a **femoral hernia** from immediately below.

The inguinal ligament must not be confused with the inguinal fold, which is the flexion crease between abdomen and leg, and runs more transversely below the ligament, medially about 2 cm and laterally 3–4 cm.

Whereas an inguinal hernia is more common in males, a femoral hernia is in females, where the often greater amounts of subcutaneous fat may make identification of the bony attachments of the inguinal ligament more difficult. Also, while a **femoral hernia appears below the inguinal ligament, it may produce swelling above the inguinal fold**.

The **inguinal ligament** runs from the **anterior superior iliac spine**, which is usually palpable (**Figure 196**), to the **pubic tubercle**, which may not be. However, the tendon of **adductor longus** runs up to the tubercle and this stands out if the leg is abducted. In a very fat person, resisted adduction from this position will help, but this is rarely necessary.

The **inguinal canal** runs from the internal inguinal ring, an opening in the transversalis fascia, to the external ring, an opening in the external oblique aponeurosis. The **internal ring** is about 2 cm above the **midpoint of the inguinal ligament** (**Figure 196**). Immediately medial to the internal ring, the **inferior epigastric artery**, a branch of the external iliac artery just before its name is changed to femoral, runs up into the abdominal wall. The arteries lie at the **mid-inguinal point**, i.e. midway between the anterior iliac spine and the symphysis pubis (hence just medial to the midpoint of the inguinal ligament). The inguinal canal runs in front of the artery to the **external ring**, some 2–3 cm above and lateral to the pubic tubercle.

1 Anterior superior iliac spine
2 Position of pubic tubercle
3 Pubic symphysis
4 Internal inguinal ring
5 External inguinal ring
6 Femoral canal ⎫
7 Femoral vein ⎬ Within the femoral sheath
8 Femoral artery ⎭
9 Femoral nerve
10 Inferior epigastric artery
11 Inguinal ligament
12 Inguinal canal

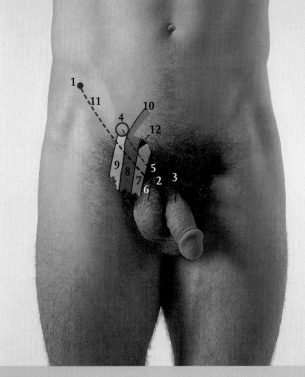

Figure 195

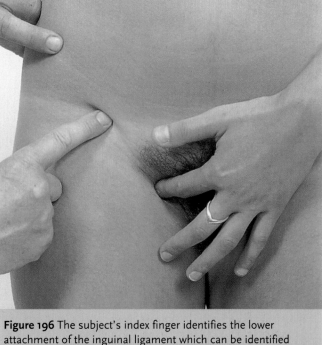

Figure 196 The subject's index finger identifies the lower attachment of the inguinal ligament which can be identified where necessary by the tendon of adductor longus. The examiner points to the midpoint of the inguinal ligament, immediately above which is the internal inguinal ring. The subject's left thumb indicates the position of the external inguinal ring.

THE EXTERNAL GENITALIA

In the female the major part of the external genital region of the perineum shows the two anteroposteriorly running **labia majora**, which run backwards from the pubic arch anteriorly, ending at the **posterior commissure**, about 2–3 cm in front of the **anus**. They are fibro-fatty cushions that carry a posterior extension of the pubic hair (**Figure 197**). Between them are the **labia minora**, much narrower folds, which may be almost totally enclosed between the labia majora or project a very variable distance below them. Anteriorly they enclose the tiny homologue of the penis, the **clitoris**, with the **urethra** opening immediately behind it. The entrance or **vestibule of the vagina** lies behind this, extending to the commissure. Although the vagina is a potentially wide canal, it is, under normal circumstances, effectively sealed. This is important because from the vagina an opening exists through the uterus and then the two uterine tubes, to the abdominal cavity, in which the ovaries lie. The labia, with mucoid secretion, give good closure externally, unless the legs are abducted quite widely. Within the vagina, the walls have transversely running folds that interlock and, with mucoid secretions, give a most effective seal.

The terms **vulva or pudendum** are given to the complete female external genitalia, which fill the anterior part of the perineum, the posterior part being the **anus**. Between the vagina and the anus is an important central tendon, firm to external pressure, the **perineal body**, which acts as a central axis for the pelvic diaphragm—the vital muscular lower wall to the pelvis and sphincteric support for the urethra and anus and, in the female, the vagina. Damage to this muscular system, as may occur in childbirth, may leave the female vulnerable to prolapse of the uterus and other problems.

In the male the **penis** is the most obvious anterior feature, hanging down from the pubis but with its root curved backwards along the perineal membrane, which gives a firm base, particularly when the organ is erected. It is covered by a loose skin that is carried down as a protective but retractile sheath over the **glans penis**, the sensitive tip to the organ. Probably for reasons of hygiene, which have become incorporated into several religious customs and social practices, the terminal sheath, the **foreskin**, is often removed (circumcision) to leave the glans permanently exposed (**Figure 198**).

The **scrotum** lies behind the penis. Embryologically this is the homologue of the labia, and the line of fusion is marked by an anteroposteriorly running ridge on the surface. The scrotum contains the **two testes and epididymes**. These, having descended into the scrotum to the cooler environment needed for **spermatogenesis**, rely on the mechanics of the scrotum for

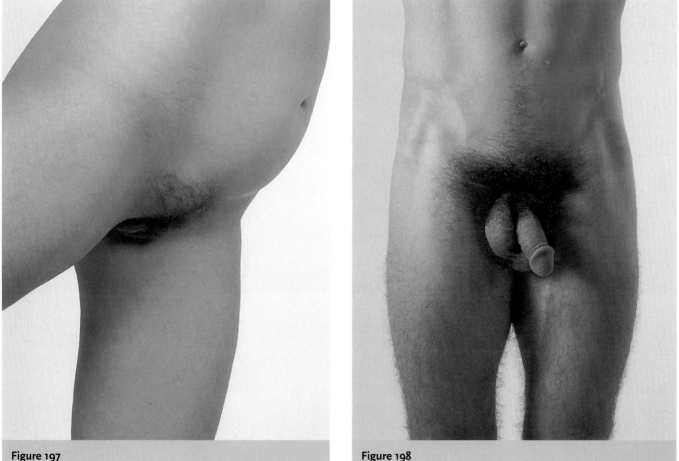

Figure 197

Figure 198

temperature control. Failure to descend, as commonly occurs, prevents spermatogenesis in that testis, even though it may be capable of producing testosterone, the male sex hormone. Usually, the left testis descends first and comes to lie lower in the scrotum than the right. Each testis hangs on a **spermatic cord**, which includes the **ductus deferens**—responsible for transferring the sperms and their containing fluid—together with the **testicular vessels and nerves**. The testis is supported by the **cremaster muscles**, lateral and (usually) medial, inserted into the root of the testicular mesentery and supplied by the genito-femoral nerve (L1–L2). In prepubertal boys the cremaster can still be highly active, but, because the processus vaginalis is closed, the testis can only be pulled up as far as the external inguinal ring; it usually comes to lie to the lateral edge of the ring, where the fascia is loosest, forming the so-called **superficial inguinal pouch**. This often gives the impression of an undescended testis unless great care is exercised in examining the boy. With the general increase in size of the genitalia at puberty, the cremaster becomes longer and much less active but still should respond to the **cremasteric reflex (L1–L2)**: if the inside of the thigh is scratched, the testis should show a degree of retraction.

The **scrotal wall** contains muscle, the **dartos**, which is involuntary and responds to temperature in a similar way to the muscle of the nipple. Its function is to maintain the testes at an even temperature, about 3°C below that of the body. It relaxes under warm conditions, taking the testes further away from body heat, and contracts when cooler (**Figures 199A&B**).

Examination of the testes should be gentle (as should all clinical examination). Pressure on the testis can be extremely painful. It is surrounded by a firm, fibrous **tunica albuginea**, and if the testis swells for any reason, the raised pressure inside the tunica produces severe pain. The **juvenile testes** are quite small; hence, if retracted by the reactive cremaster muscles, they can easily be lost to the examiner, in the inguinal tissues. In the **adult** they are 4–5 cm in height and 3 cm in diameter, with the comma-shaped collection of tubules—the **epididymis**—around the posterior aspect and leading off to the ductus deferens. In the neck of the scrotum, above the level of the testis, the cord can be felt as an indistinct structure, though the **ductus deferens** is easy to feel, owing to its very thick muscular wall, as a firm round cord.

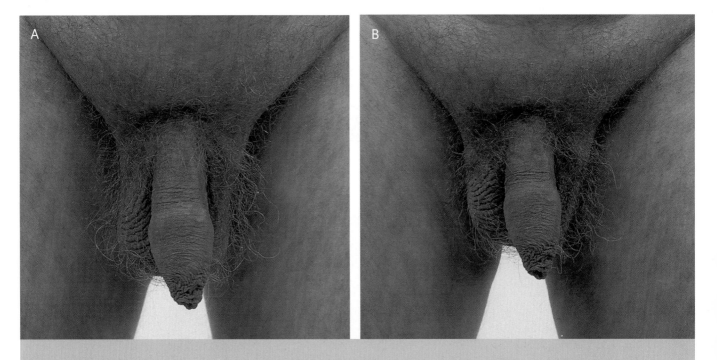

Figure 199A and B The uncircumcised penis and scrotum in moderate temperature conditions (**A**) and showing some degree of contraction of the scrotal wall on cooling (**B**). Note that even the size of the penis is much influenced by temperature, as is to be expected in a highly vascular organ.

NERVES OF THE THORACIC AND ABDOMINAL WALLS

The general innervation comes from the **segmental spinal nerves**. The **posterior primary rami** innervate the erector spinae muscles and provide sensory supply to the overlying skin, mainly as far as the outer edge of the muscles, but some overlap with the anterior primary rami may extend as far as the posterior axillary line. The **anterior primary rami** of C5–T1 join the **brachial plexus** to innervate the arm, and those in the **lumbosacral** outflow go to the leg; none goes to the trunk. Thus, C4 gives cutaneous innervation to the shoulder and clavicular regions, to be succeeded on the chest by T2 in a segmental band. Similarly there is a jump from upper lumbar to lower sacral in the perineal region. In the thorax the segmental nerves run around the chest wall in the intercostal spaces, supplying thoracic wall musculature and giving cutaneous branches (**Figure 200**). A major **lateral branch** comes through in the mid-axillary line, to give a posterior and a larger anterior division. The posterior division supplies the lateral aspect of the back, and the anterior, the anterolateral aspect of the trunk. The lower six thoracic and L1 run down to supply the anterolateral aspect of the abdominal wall, though T12 and L1 give little supply to the flank but run down to the gluteal region over the hip.

The main nerves then continue to the front of the trunk, giving terminal sensory branches to the skin. The **lower six thoracic and first lumbar supply the abdominal musculature** and the overlying skin. L1 divides early into **iliohypogastric and ilio-inguinal branches**. The former supplies skin around the pubis; the latter runs through the inguinal canal (or alongside it), supplying skin of the medial part of the groin and the anterior parts of the penis and scrotum (in a male) or the clitoris and labia (in a female). This root also supplies the lowest part of the internal oblique and transversus abdominis muscles and its loss, as at surgery, may predispose to an inguinal hernia due to the reduced motor control over that component of the muscles covering the inguinal canal. **T10 gives segmental supply to the umbilicus (Figure 200)**.

Each segmental nerve will usually supply its own segment and overlap into those immediately above and below, and some even to the ones above and below those. Thus, loss of an individual segmental nerve, as after an abdominal operation, usually—but not always—passes unnoticed.

The roots of the penis or clitoris and the anterior parts of the scrotum or labia majora receive sensory innervation from the ilio-inguinal (L1) and genitofemoral (L1–L2) nerves, but, immediately behind, the innervation changes to S2–S4 from the pudendal nerves. These latter supply the major part of the skin of the penis or clitoris, and the external genital and anal regions. A **low spinal anaesthetic block** gives excellent control for much of the perineal region, but care must be taken not to move too far anteriorly, where the region supplied by L1–L2 will not be anaesthetised.

Local **anaesthetic block of the intercostal nerves** may be called for. The main nerve runs along the lower border of the rib. If the injection is made posteriorly near the angle of the rib (avoiding the lung), the anaesthetic will travel up and down in the paravertebral gutter for a segment or two, giving a wider area of anaesthesia from a single injection, either for the chest wall or, in the lower nerves, for abdominal surgery (though muscular relaxation may be poor).

REFERRED PAIN

Most deep structures, particularly in the thorax and abdomen, have poor sensory localisation. Deep sensation lacks the various localised sensory modalities available from the skin, though pain from locomotor structures may be localised. From the viscera, even that localisation is missing and pain may be referred to a superficial region away from the original site (**Figure 201**). Pain from the **heart or bronchi** (the lungs and visceral pleura are insensitive unless the parietal pleura is involved) tends to be diffusely concentrated to the sternum. Pain from the **diaphragm and the related pericardium** may be

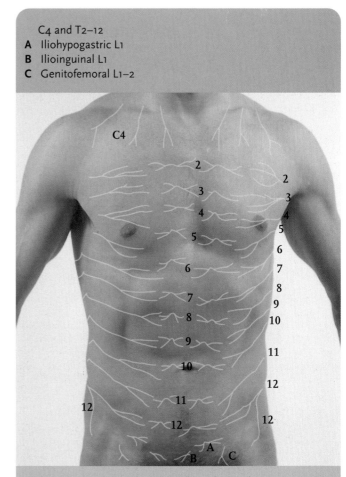

C4 and T2–12
A Iliohypogastric L1
B Ilioinguinal L1
C Genitofemoral L1–2

Figure 200 Cutaneous nerve supply to the trunk.

referred to the C4 (and C5) skin areas shared with the diaphragm: the shoulder (C4) and down the arm (C5). Pain in these regions on the left side may be of cardiac origin if associated with sternal pain. Pain of **angina pectoris** (i.e. true heart pain) may also appear as a 'crushing' pain to the left side of the sternum and may spread down the medial side of the arm (T1–T5).

In the abdomen, pain from the viscera tends to be localised to the midline. The **stomach and upper abdominal** structures are referred centrally to the epigastrium, but an indication to left or right may come from the stomach or liver and gall-bladder. Hypersensitivity or pain from these structures may also affect the area below the scapula, to left or right. The **intestines** refer generally to the umbilical region, with the **transverse and descending colons** centrally but below. If, however, inflammation etc. affects the parietal peritoneum (or the parietal pleura in the chest), then localisation is good, as surface nerves become involved. Thus, the characteristic pain of **appendicitis** is initially to the umbilicus, as a dull ache, but later, inflammation may affect the overlying peritoneum in the right iliac fossa, where the pain becomes sharper and localised (though in a retrocaecal appendix the localisation may be less obvious).

Pain from the **kidneys** may be referred to the loins as a dull ache, but where the **renal pelvis or ureter** is affected it becomes more localised to the inguinal region. The **pelvic organs**, including the bladder, generally give suprapubic pain.

Although the pain does not originate in the referred area, it often exhibits hypersensitivity and may even become redder. The pain may also be obliterated by local anaesthesia of the referred area.

BLOOD VESSELS OF THE THORACIC AND ABDOMINAL WALLS

The body wall receives a good blood supply with anastomoses between dorsal and ventral systems, which can often help in providing alternative routes if the axial vessels to the arms or legs are lost proximally.

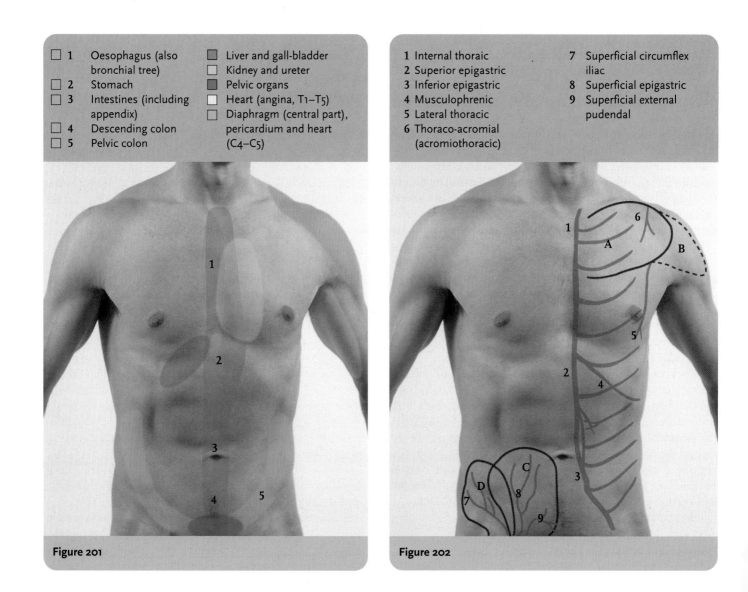

☐ 1 Oesophagus (also bronchial tree)
☐ 2 Stomach
☐ 3 Intestines (including appendix)
☐ 4 Descending colon
☐ 5 Pelvic colon
☐ Liver and gall-bladder
☐ Kidney and ureter
☐ Pelvic organs
☐ Heart (angina, T1–T5)
☐ Diaphragm (central part), pericardium and heart (C4–C5)

1 Internal thoracic
2 Superior epigastric
3 Inferior epigastric
4 Musculophrenic
5 Lateral thoracic
6 Thoraco-acromial (acromiothoracic)
7 Superficial circumflex iliac
8 Superficial epigastric
9 Superficial external pudendal

Figure 201

Figure 202

Dorsal supply comes from the aorta, which gives intercostal arteries, running around the lower borders of the ribs in the intercostal spaces, and lumbar arteries below them. Anterior intersegmental arteries arise from the main limb arteries. **Thoracic branches of the axillary and subclavian arteries give anterior and lateral supply** to anastomose with the intercostal arteries (**Figure 202**). Anteriorly the **internal thoracic (mammary) artery** runs down from about 2 cm above the medial end of the clavicle inside the chest wall, 1–1.5 cm out from the sternal border, anastomosing directly with the intercostal arteries, which therefore have anterior and posterior supplies. It also gives a major supply to the breast. It continues into the abdomen to become the **superior epigastric artery**. This runs down in the rectus sheath behind the muscle, maintaining the anastomoses with the intercostal arteries, before entering and supplying the rectus muscle and anastomosing with the inferior epigastric artery.

The **inferior epigastric artery** comes from the external iliac vessel, passes up medial to the deep inguinal ring and then to the rectus abdominis muscle, and anastomoses with the lower intercostal and the superior epigastric arteries. The **deep circumflex artery** also runs from the external iliac to the lower abdominal wall and anastomoses with gluteal arteries. Slightly more distally, the femoral artery gives **superficial epigastric and circumflex iliac arteries** (as well as pudendal). These originate about 1 cm below the inguinal ligament and run up to supply the lower abdominal wall.

The **veins** follow essentially the same routes, with the posterior azygos system acting alongside the aorta in the thorax.

AXIAL VASCULAR FLAPS

The rich anastomoses offer excellent opportunities for axial vascular skin flaps to be prepared when needed for repair (also myocutaneous flaps based on the vascular pedicle of muscle, e.g. pectoralis and latissimus dorsi, as well as fasciocutaneous flaps). An excellent long cutaneous flap can be raised on the

upper perforating arteries from the internal thoracic artery and running out towards the deltoid region—a **deltopectoral flap (Figure 202, see A)** With possible extension to **B** after thorraco-acromial division and delay, it can give good, soft and thin skin cover for either the face or neck.

The **superficial epigastric**,(C), and **circumflex iliac**,(D), vessels give good axes for the transfer of lower abdominal skin, e.g. for repair of a hand or elsewhere as a free flap. The skin is good, but the superficial epigastric includes pubic hair.

SUPERFICIAL FEATURES OF THE ANTERIOR ABDOMINAL WALL

Other than hair-bearing areas, the **umbilicus** is an obvious feature (**Figure 203**): extremely variable in form and even position, being a scar of the umbilical cord and its contents. The bladder always retains a link, the median umbilical ligament, which is why stimulation of the umbilicus may have its T10 sensory response supplemented by a diffuse supra-umbilical sensation, characteristic of the bladder. The **umbilicus** is usually level with L3 vertebral spine but may even be as low as L5 in a stocky individual with a protuberant abdomen.

The **bony landmarks of the abdomen** are at the upper and lower limits: the xiphisternum and the costal margins above; the pubis below, with the ilia laterally. The **anterior superior iliac spines** are usually obvious (see **Figure 195**), from which the **iliac crest** curves upwards and backwards with a lateral flare, which is usually more obvious in the broader pelvis of a female. About 5 cm behind the anterior spine, a prominence—the **tubercle**—may be palpable in a slim person. A similar distance behind this, the ilium reaches its **crest**.

In a reasonably slim, muscular person, the midline **linea alba** may be seen and, particularly if the rectus is contracted, its lateral border, the **linea semilunaris**, the **fibrous intersections** in the muscle and also the anterior limits of the musculature of the external oblique (see **Figure 191**, page 94).

In view of the relatively featureless expanse of the abdomen, a number of planes are described to help delineate, of which the **transpyloric plane** is important. Originally described as midway between the suprasternal notch and the upper border of the pubis, a more practical clinical level is midway between the xiphisternum and the (albeit variable) umbilicus (**Figure 204**), or a patient's hand breadth below the xiphisternal joint. The plane is also at the level where the linea semilunaris meets the costal margin, at the tip of the ninth costal cartilage. Posteriorly it is at the level of the lower border of L1 vertebra and its spine.

The plane may only be transpyloric when a person is supine; when standing, the pylorus may be 3–10 cm below. The level is helpful in identifying the positions of several other structures. The **gall-bladder** normally lies behind the tip of the ninth costal cartilage. The **renal vessels** link the hila of the kidneys with the aorta and the inferior vena cava, though the kidneys, like the stomach, drop in upright posture. The **superior mesenteric artery** leaves the aorta at this level and also the **portal vein** is formed. Some 3–5 cm to the right of the

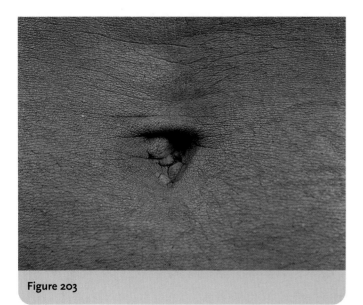

Figure 203

midline is the **aditus to the lesser sac of peritoneum** and in front of that the hepatic vessels and the common bile duct run in the free edge of the lesser omentum.

Other useful levels are:

Xiphisternum—body of T11 (spine of T10).

Iliac crests (supracristal plane)—L4 spinous process.

Iliac tubercles (intertubercular plane)—L5 spinous process.

Anterior and posterior superior iliac spines—S2.

Upper border of symphysis pubis (and centre of the acetabulum)—tip of coccyx (in a female); tip of sacrum (in a male).

A subcostal plane is sometimes described (i.e. tenth costal cartilage) but this varies, not only with build but also with posture and state of respiration. It is, however, usually at L3 (and the umbilicus) when the person is relaxed and lying supine.

By using the transverse lines of the transpyloric and intertubercular planes, with vertical ones drawn down from the middle of the clavicles to the mid-inguinal point (see page 96), the abdominal and lower thoracic walls can be divided into regions, to facilitate clinical description (**Figure 205**).

THE VISCERA

The position and shape of some viscera vary with posture, state of respiration, the physiological state of the organ and the functional control of the abdominal wall. These factors must be considered before accepting evidence of pathology.

The position of viscera relative to posture depends not only upon gravity but also to a major extent upon the physical state and tonus of the anterior abdominal wall. The **stomach** at its cardiac end moves to a great extent with the diaphragm in respiration, but the pylorus, while possibly being at the transpyloric plane when supine, may descend by two vertebrae or 3–10 cm in upright posture. The **kidneys** are usually described as having an acceptable descent of up to 6 cm, but even greater levels of descent have been recorded in perfectly healthy medical students. Upright posture affects the **transverse colon**, but even retroperitoneal structures such as the **pancreas** and **duodenum** are affected to some extent. The range of movement may be limited by vascular attachments, e.g. the **liver**, which moves with respiration and the diaphragm, but is firmly related to the inferior vena cava, which in turn is linked to the central tendon of the diaphragm. The **spleen**, which moves with respiration and becomes more vertical in upright posture, is nevertheless limited in its range by vascular attachments. So also are the kidneys, for although

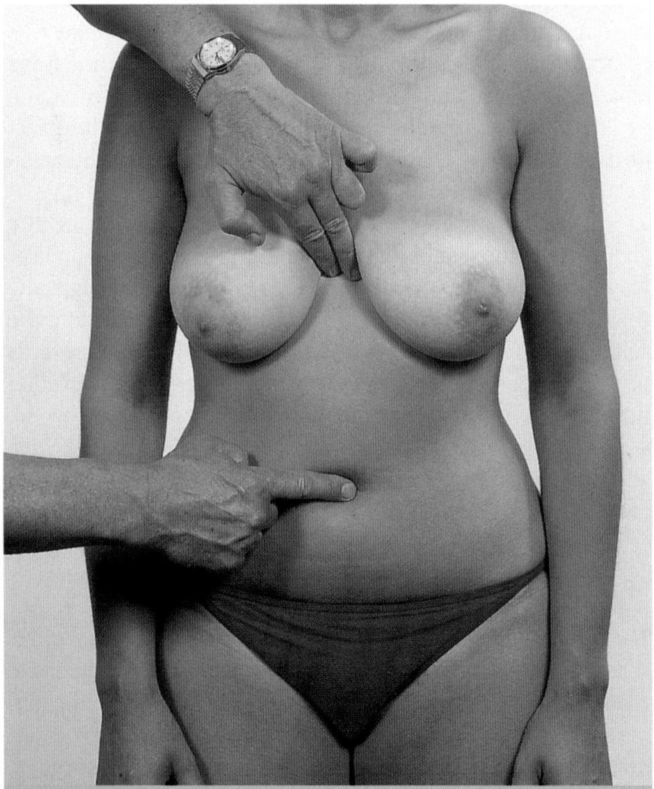

1 Right hypochondrium	A Midclavicular line
2 Right lumbar	B Transpyloric plane
3 Right iliac	C Transtubercular plane
4 Left hypochondrium	D Subcostal plane
5 Left lumbar	E Supracristal plane
6 Left iliac	F Interspinous plane
7 Epigastrium	
8 Umbilical	
9 Hypogastrium	

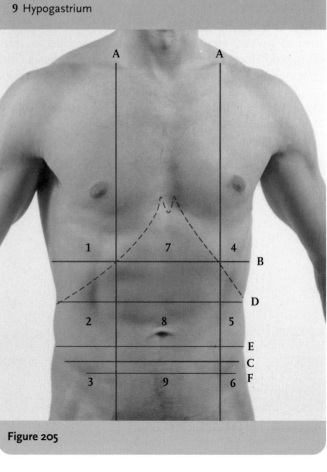

Figure 204

Figure 205

they descend to a considerable distance, further drop is limited by the vessels and if movement is too free, their vascular supply can be affected.

The positions of the liver, gallbladder, spleen and kidneys are markedly affected by the descent of the diaphragm in deep inspiration, and this movement is made use of in their clinical examination by palpation.

The liver lies largely in the right hypogastrium and extends across the epigastrium. Although the liver is described anatomically as having right and left lobes with intervening caudate and quadrate lobes, the intervening lobes form part of the functional left lobe. They divide the liver through the gallbladder at the front to the inferior vena cava behind. Seen from the surface by a line drawn up from the tip of the ninth costal cartilage to the level of the diaphragm, they form the upper surface of the liver (**Figure 206**).

The liver moves with the diaphragm in respiration (**Figure 206**) and, as maximal diaphragmatic movement is related to the crura, the anterior margin of the liver moves to the right in inspiration. On the right the upper surface of the liver follows the right dome of the diaphragm so that in quiet respiration it reaches the level of the fifth costal cartilage (or in the midclavicular line the fourth intercostal space). The line then runs across the xiphisternal joint to the level of the sixth costal cartilage on the left. The lower margin follows the costal margin on the right and then crosses the epigastrium from the tip of the ninth right costal cartilage to the eighth costal cartilage on

the left, continues upwards inside the costal margin and ends level with the xiphisternal joint 8–10 cm from the midline. In deep expiration the liver rises, whereas in full inspiration its anterior margin projects beyond the costal margin on the right, but not usually to an extent that is palpable. Although the liver lies in the epigastrium, even here it is not normally palpable.

Direct **clinical examination of the liver** is limited by its being covered by the rib cage. As the liver is solid, percussion gives an area of dullness compared with the resonant lung above and the other abdominal contents below, but the upper margin is masked by the overlying lung. Pathological enlargement may project the anterior margin below the rib cage, especially on inspiration. If the fingers are laid parallel with the costal margin, over the relaxed abdomen, and the patient asked to breathe deeply, the lower sharp margin may be felt moving across the fingers (**Figure 207**).

Liver biopsy is a common clinical examination. If the patient is asked to breathe out, the biopsy needle can be passed through the lower intercostal space in the midclavicular line, without puncturing the lung.

The gallbladder normally lies behind the tip of the ninth costal cartilage, i.e. where the lateral margin of rectus abdominis joins the costal margin, and at the transpyloric plane. Normally it is impalpable, even when pathological. However, if the fingers are pressed in below the ninth costal margin (as in **Figure 207**) and the patient asked to breathe in, pain may be induced from a diseased gallbladder, commonly producing a 'catch' in the breath.

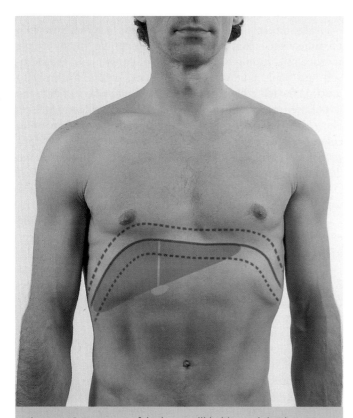

Figure 206 Positions of the liver, gallbladder and diaphram.

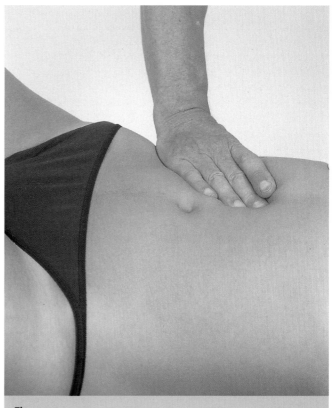

Figure 207

The **stomach** lies in the left hypochondrial, epigastric (mainly) and umbilical regions. It is subject to numerous variations in shape and position (**Figure 208**). The **oesophagus** penetrates the diaphragm about 3 cm to the left of the midline at the level of T10; or behind the upper part of the sixth costal cartilage, becoming the stomach behind the seventh cartilage. On the right the line of the oesophagus continues, curving to the right, as the **lesser curvature of the stomach**, to the **pylorus**, which lies some 1–2 cm to the right of the midline, at or about the transpyloric plane, if the person is supine and the stomach empty. The left border bulges upwards to form the usually gas-filled **fundus**, which rises as high as the fifth rib in the midclavicular line. The **greater curvature** follows a very variable course to the pylorus, depending upon the position, build and muscular state of the individual and contents of the stomach and of other viscera. The pylorus may drop 3–10 cm in upright posture and the lower margin of the greater curvature, i.e. the pyloric antrum, may descend even more—particularly when full, in a slimly built asthenic individual—to well below the umbilicus and into the false pelvis. In a broadly built person the stomach tends to lie more transversely and have the so-called steerhorn shape, whereas the slim asthenic person is likely to have a J-shaped structure.

Because of its soft nature, even when full, the stomach is normally difficult to feel. Occasionally the pylorus is hypertrophied in a young infant, when it may be felt as a hard lump, particularly on inspiration. The stomach commonly exhibits a high-pitched resonance to percussion, though this is largely lost after feeding and it is often difficult to differentiate the stomach resonance from that of the underlying transverse colon.

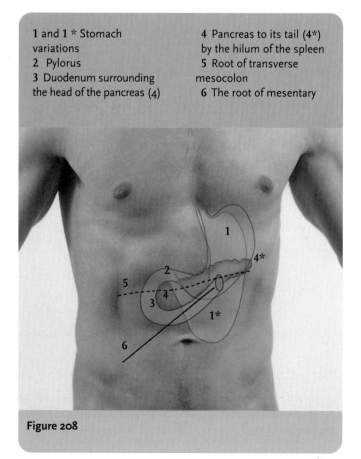

1 and 1 * Stomach variations	4 Pancreas to its tail (4*) by the hilum of the spleen
2 Pylorus	5 Root of transverse mesocolon
3 Duodenum surrounding the head of the pancreas (4)	6 The root of mesentery

Figure 208

THE INTESTINES

The duodenum continues from the stomach and curves around the head of the pancreas (**Figure 208**). Its first 2–3 cm is carried on a mesentery and therefore exhibits the mobility of the pylorus, but the second half of the transversely running first part becomes retroperitoneal and more fixed, roughly in the transpyloric plane or a little above. About 5 cm to the right of the midline, the second part runs vertically downwards for 7–8 cm before turning at right angles to the left, about level with the costal margin (L3). The third part of the duodenum crosses the midline more or less horizontally, and about 1–2 cm to the left it turns slightly upwards to the duodenojejunal junction, about 3cm to the left of the midline in the transpyloric plane. The junction is fairly stable, held by the suspensory ligament of the duodenum (Treitz).

The remaining components of the small intestine—the **jejunum** and the **ileum**—form a long twisting tube that packs much of the abdomen and pelvis. It is maintained on a mesentery, the root of which runs obliquely downwards and to the right, from the duodenojejunal junction to the caecum, i.e. towards the anterior superior iliac spine (**Figure 208**).

The caecum lies in the roughly triangular area bounded by the intertubercular line and the lateral ¹/₂ of the inguinal ligament (**Figure 209**).

The appendix is so variable that the position of its origin is the only reasonable surface marking, i.e. at McBurney's point, at the junction of the middle and lower thirds of the line joining the umbilicus with the anterior superior iliac spine (**Figure 209**).

The ascending colon lies in the right flank and is usually impalpable (**Figure 209**). It ascends roughly to the level of the ninth intercostal space, under cover of the liver, i.e. just below the transpyloric plane. At the **hepatic flexure** it turns into the **transverse colon**, crossing the abdomen on the transverse mesocolon, looping below the greater curvature of the stomach and usually below the umbilicus, before running up towards the **left (splenic) flexure**. This lies some 10 cm to the left of the midline and behind the eighth costal cartilage, i.e. above the transpyloric plane. The root of the **transverse mesocolon (Figure 208)** can be indicated by a line linking the right 10th costal cartilage with the left eighth. From this region the **descending colon** runs down in the flank inside the ilium. It can often be felt due to its contained faeces, if the abdominal wall is relaxed.

NB If the patient is tense when the abdomen is being examined, its wall can often be relaxed by bending up the legs at the hips and knees.

The pelvic colon runs on a mesentery **(Figure 209)** that forms an inverted 'V', running up from the level of the left inguinal ligament to the sacral promontory and then down in the midline to 2–3 cm below the anterior superior iliac spines, when the midline **rectum** begins, i.e. at S3.

The pancreas lies with its head to the right of the midline, within the curve of the duodenum. Its neck overlies the aorta and the superior mesenteric artery and thus is in the midline of the body. Its body and tail go upwards and to the left. The tail approaches the hilum of the spleen roughly in the midclavicular line, a little above the transpyloric plane (**Figure 208**).

1 Anterior superior iliac
   spine
2 Tubercle of ilium
3 Crest of ilium
4 Line of inguinal ligament
5 Caecum
6 Root of appendix
   (McBurney's point)
7 Ascending colon
8 Transverse colon
9 Descending colon
10 Pelvic colon
11 Root of pelvic mesocolon

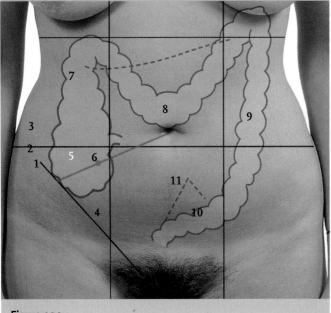

Figure 209

1 Bladder empty
2 Bladder moderately
   distended
3 Uterus with empty
   bladder
4 Uterine tube
5 Ovary
6 Kidney
7 Ureter
8 Pancreas
9 Duodenum

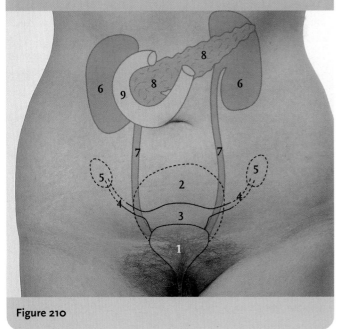

Figure 210

The spleen lies above the left kidney and behind the stomach, between it and the diaphragm posteriorly, being between the ninth and eleventh ribs and along the axis of the tenth, from the lateral border of the erector spinae to the midaxillary line. Although it is on the posterolateral chest wall, it is separated from it by the diaphragm and pleura. It is vulnerable to injury from the back. In deep inspiration the lungs give it some protection. In quiet respiration the spleen can be delineated by percussion. It can only be projected against the fingers, below the left anterior costal margin on inspiration, if considerably enlarged.

The kidneys lie on the posterior abdominal wall (**Figure 210**), on either side of the vertebrae, their hila projecting anteromedially. Each kidney has a height of 11 cm and the two hila are 4–5 cm from the midline. When lying supine the hila of the kidneys should be around the transpyloric plane, the right kidney lower than the left, so that the transpyloric plane cuts the upper part of the right hilum and the lower part of the left. From the back the lower poles of the kidneys should be about 3–4 cm above the iliac crests and the upper parts deep to the lowest two ribs. In upright posture the kidneys may drop up to 6 cm and even greater descent may be found on occasions, without obvious pathology.

In a slim individual lying supine, the lower pole of the normal kidney may be felt descending on inspiration, if one hand is pushed forwards from the loin and the other presses into the flank. Enlarged kidneys may be felt more easily (**Figure 211**).

The suprarenal glands lie above the kidneys and their lower aspects may be estimated as being about 5 cm above the transpyloric plane and on each side of the vertebrae.

The ureters leave the kidneys at the hila and run down to the back of the bladder. In the supine position they can be

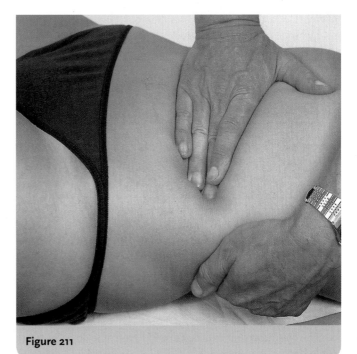

Figure 211

delineated as running downwards from the transpyloric plane at 5 cm from the midline. Initially they run almost vertically, but then curve medially to enter the bladder behind and a little medial to the pubic tubercles. In their course down, they cross the sacro-iliac joints and the common iliac arteries at their bifurcation, which is at the intertubercular line about 4 cm from the midline.

The bladder lies largely behind and a little above the pubis when empty. It then has an essentially flat upper surface, covered by intestine and, in a female, the body of the uterus. As if fills it becomes more dome-shaped and a normally filled bladder extends upwards to about midway between the pubis and the umbilicus (**Figure 210**). In retention of urine it can reach the umbilicus or even higher. In a baby it lies entirely within the abdomen and has a more tubular shape, only reaching adult form and position in late childhood.

The bladder is normally impalpable, but where it extends above the pubis its upper border can usually be delineated by percussion.

In a male the **prostate** lies below the bladder in a retropubic position, where it can be examined rectally. It measures 3.5–4 cm in diameter, has a firm consistency and its right and left lobes are divided by a shallow groove.

The uterus in an adult female lies behind and above the bladder. When the bladder is empty the uterus projects only a short distance above the pubis. As the bladder fills, the normal anteverted uterus is pushed more vertically so that it projects well above the pubis, as do the uterine tubes (**Figure 210**). During pregnancy it enlarges enormously and extends up towards the costal margins, pushing the other viscera ahead. During the second half of pregnancy, but not otherwise, the uterus is easy to feel from the abdomen. However, it is possible to examine it vaginally, pressing it forwards from the cervix against a second hand placed above the pubis. After childbearing the uterus remains a little enlarged and never returns fully to its original size.

The ovaries lie roughly level with the anterior superior iliac spines, above the mid-inguinal point, though these are also pulled up by the uterus in pregnancy.

THE GREAT VESSELS

The aorta enters the abdomen in the midline, in front of the body of T12, i.e. about 3–4 cm above the transpyloric plane (see page 102). It runs down in the midline to end slightly to the left by dividing in front of L4 (intercristal plane), into the common iliac arteries. Within the abdomen it is around 10 cm long. The **coeliac axis** leaves immediately after the aorta has entered the abdomen (T12), dividing almost immediately into hepatic, splenic and left gastric branches. The **superior mesenteric artery** is given off at or a little above the transpyloric plane, where the **renal arteries** also leave. Slightly below, the **gonadic vessels** leave, followed by the **inferior mesenteric** at approximately L3, i.e. the subcostal plane and at the level of the umbilicus.

The common iliac arteries diverge from the aorta in front of the body of L4, and each divides into **internal and external**

branches at the sacro-iliac joints, in the intertubercular plane about 4 cm from the midline. From here the **external iliac arteries** run around the pelvis, each leaving under the middle of the inguinal ligament to become a **femoral artery**.

The **inferior vena cava** is formed in front of L5 by union of the **common iliac veins**. It thus begins at the intertubercular plane some 2–3 cm to the right of the midline and runs upwards, parallel to the vertebral bodies, to pass through the central tendon of the diaphragm at the level of the xiphisternal joint (T8–T9).

The **portal vein** is formed behind the neck of the pancreas by union of the **superior mesenteric and splenic veins**, roughly in the midline and about 1–2 cm below the transpyloric plane, from which position it runs up to the liver.

The abdominal lymphatics generally follow the aorta and therefore can be grouped with this. Those from the viscera form upon its anterior aspect, with the body-wall lymphatics along its sides.

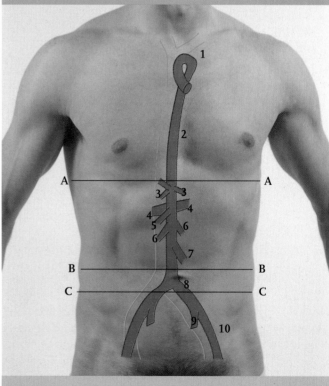

A Transpyloric plane (L1–L2)	**5** Superior mesenteric
B Intercristal plane	**6** Gonadal
C Intertubercular plane (L5)	**7** Inferior mesenteric
1 Arch of aorta	**8** Common iliac
2 Descending aorta	**9** Internal iliac
3 Coeliac axis (T12)	**10** External iliac
4 Renal arteries	

Figure 212 The levels of the brachiocephalic veins and the superior vena cava are shown, as are the common iliac veins with the inferior vena cava.

Chapter 10

The legs

BONY LANDMARKS AROUND THE HIP

The **anterior superior iliac spine** is usually readily palpable, as is the **greater trochanter** of the femur. The **pubis** may be difficult to feel—particularly in a female, being overlaid by the mons pubis (veneris)—but its tubercle can easily be identified by running a finger along the tensed adductor longus tendon (see page 96). In normal stance the anterior superior iliac spine should lie in the same vertical plane as the symphysis pubis and on the same horizontal plane as the posterior superior iliac spine and S2 vertebra. The upper aspect of the pubis should be at the same level as the tip of the coccyx in a female and the tip of the sacrum in a male. (The difference is due to the sacrum being shorter and broader in the female.) The top of the greater trochanter is at the same level.

The **greater trochanter** produces a surface prominence, particularly in a slim male. In normal posture the neck of the femur runs a little backwards. (In a radiograph the neck of the femur is shown best by turning the leg inwards, whereas to show the lesser trochanter, which lies behind and medially, the leg should be turned laterally.) The top of the greater trochanter should be level with, but behind, the centre of the hip joint. By pressing upwards into the buttock, the **ischial tuberosity** should be palpable when the gluteal muscles are relaxed.

Any **difference between leg length** is clinically important, as is the site of shortening. A line drawn across the two anterior superior iliac spines should be parallel with one drawn across the two greater trochanters and, with the person standing, both should be level (**Figure 213**).

If, on standing, the anterior superior iliac spines are not at the same level, a measure should be made from them to the tip of the medial malleoli. If there is shortening on one side and the lines between the spines and trochanters are parallel, then the shortening will be below that level. Measurements should then be made of the spines to the knee, taking the top of the tibial table on the medial side of the patella or the tibial tubercle, and from there to the medial malleolus. A slight difference in leg length is quite common.

The hip joint is an extremely stable ball-and-socket joint, but has good movement on what, ideally, is a stable pelvis. Ranges at the hip can appear greater due to movement in the lumbar spine and this must be excluded in clinical examination of the joint. Movements available are flexion, extension, abduction, adduction, medial and lateral rotation and their combination, and circumduction.

Flexion should be examined with the knee bent to prevent tension in the hamstrings. The range can appear to allow the thigh to reach the abdominal wall but part of this comes from

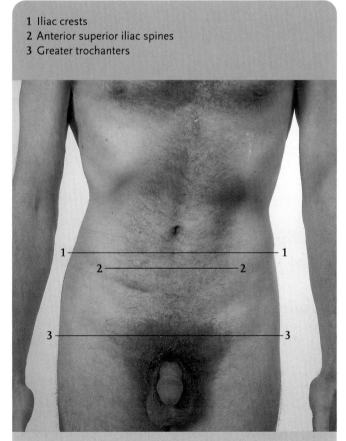

1 Iliac crests
2 Anterior superior iliac spines
3 Greater trochanters

Figure 213 From this stance it appears at first sight that one leg is longer than the other, but the anterior superior spines are level. The problem is one of mild scoliosis.

lumbar flexion. If the examiner's hand is placed under the hollow of the person's back as the hip is flexed, it can check when lumbar flexion begins, at the end of the normal hip range—about 120° (**Figure 214A**).

Extension is normally limited to 15–20° but can appear much more, as in the arabesque of classical ballet, where the leg can be carried quite high to the back, by extension of the lumbar spine (see **Figure 194** page 95). To test, the person should lie face down (prone), and the leg to be inspected lifted by the examiner, the weight of the leg remaining on the couch being used to limit lumbar extension (**Figure 214B**).

Abduction and adduction can be examined with the subject supine. The straight leg is carried to the side, watching the anterior superior iliac spines for signs of movement, which occurs at the limit of hip abduction; then taken across the other leg into adduction. Abduction is possible to 45–60° and adduction to about 45°, though here the movement is limited by the other leg. It is important that no rotation be allowed in the leg because **lateral rotation increases the range of abduction**, a phenomenon used in classical ballet, where 'turn-out' at the hips greatly increases the lateral freedom of the legs (**Figure 216**).

Medial and lateral rotation can be examined with the person lying prone. If the knee is bent to 90° and the thigh rotated, the lower leg can be used as an indicator of the degree of rotation—normally about 60–70° each way (**Figure 215**). Sometimes it is useful to examine the ranges with the hips flexed. With the

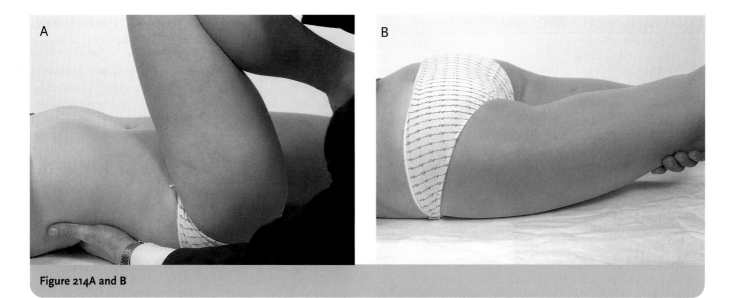

Figure 214A and B

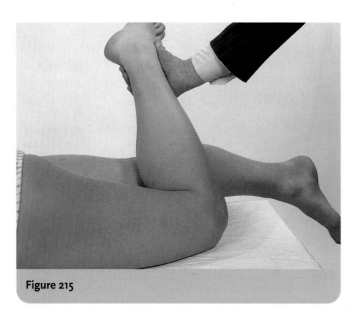

Figure 215

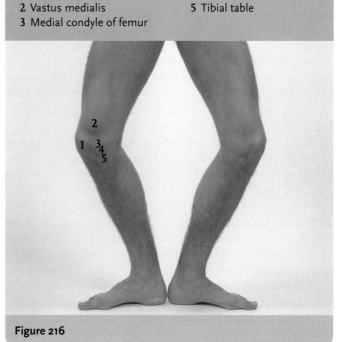

1 Patella
2 Vastus medialis
3 Medial condyle of femur
4 Joint space
5 Tibial table

Figure 216

person sitting, the leg can be swung each way, or the manoeuvre can be carried out with the person supine, with the hip and knee bent to 90°.

1 Patella
2 Tubercle of tibia
3 Tibial condyle
4 Head of fibula
5 Joint space
6 Biceps femoris
7 Iliotibial tract
8 Vastus lateralis
9 Rectus femoris

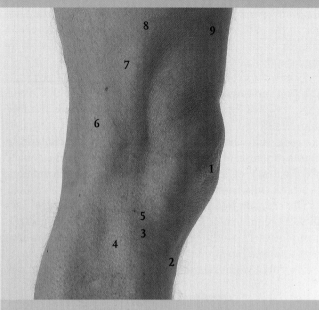

Figure 217 Lateral side of the knee

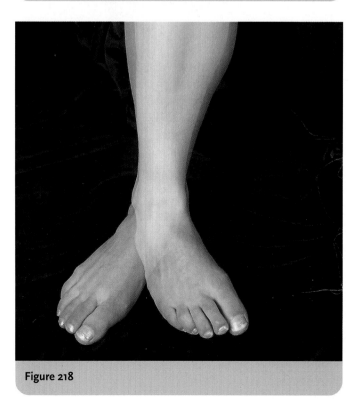

Figure 218

BONY POINTS AROUND THE KNEE

The **patella** is the most obvious feature of the knee in a slim person. In a muscular male the vastus medialis may mask the upper part of its medial edge, but the lower part and its lateral edge are obvious, the belly of vastus lateralis ending much higher than the medialis. In a fat person the central part of the patella should be palpable. The patella lies on the lower anterior surface of the femur when the knee is straight and moves around its distal end as the joint bends. Thus, when kneeling, the femur transmits the load of the body through the patella.

If the quadriceps muscles are relaxed, the patella can be moved medially and laterally to some extent, though lateral movement is limited by the anterior prominence of the **lateral femoral condyle**, which can be felt projecting deep to the lateral edge of the patella. This lateral bony prominence plays some part, with the medial pull of vastus medialis, in preventing lateral dislocation of the patella, due to the angulated knee, a risk greater in females because of the wider pelvis and greater angulation (**Figure 220**).

Below the patella and joined to it by the **ligamentum patellae** is the **tibial tuberosity**, an anterior prominence on the upper end of the tibia. The tendon is inserted into the lower part of the tuberosity, which has a smoother upper part that is separated from the tendon by the **deep infrapatellar bursa**. A **superficial infrapatellar bursa** allows the skin to move freely over the tuberosity, as a **prepatellar bursa** acts likewise for the patella.

Above the tibial tuberosity and to each side of the ligamentum patellae is a hollow where the joint space can be felt, above the sharp edges of the **tibial condyles**. The space behind the ligamentum patellae is filled by soft fat (which pushes folds of synovium into the joint space between the femoral condyles, the alar folds). Lateral to the fat, the anterior horns of the **menisci** can be felt, more easily in the extended knee, when they tend to project a little.

The space of the knee joint can be followed around the sides until, medially, its detail is reduced by the broad **medial collateral ligament** and the overlying tendons (**Figure 216**). Laterally the **iliotibial tract** has a similar effect with the knee in extension (**Figure 217**), but in flexion the space can be felt, crossed by the rounded cord of the **lateral collateral ligament**, running from the lateral femoral condyle to the head of the fibula. In extension this ligament is overlaid by the tendon of **biceps femoris**.

Above the joint space the **medial and lateral epicondyles of the femur** form projections, while on the medial side the tendon of insertion of adductor magnus leads to the **adductor tubercle**. Below the joint the **medial condyle of the tibia** continues downwards into its subcutaneous surface, the shin. The **lateral tibial condyle** is overlaid by the prominent head of the **fibula**. Posteriorly the condyles of the femur are covered by muscle masses of gastrocnemius and the hamstrings, leaving a hollow between: the fat-filled popliteal fossa.

MOVEMENT AT THE KNEE

The knee is often considered as a simple hinge joint, but accessory movements are of functional and clinical importance. **Flexion** can bring the calf into contact with the back of the thigh, but this may not be achieved as an active movement with the hip extended, because of the active insufficiency of the flexor muscles. **Extension** should be to a full 180° but is commonly more in loose-limbed individuals, who may well be capable of 15–20° beyond this: the so-called **sway-back knee**.

Rotation is an important accessory movement at the knee, being at its greatest at about 60° of flexion (**Figure 218**), the range reducing until at full extension even passive rotation should be impossible. However, as the knee is taken into full extension a small amount of active lateral rotation of the tibia on the femur takes place, **'locking' the knee** into a stable close-packed state for standing, with tightening of the cruciate ligaments. On the initiation of flexion the process is reversed: the tibia is rotated medially on the femur by the activity of **popliteus**, a flexor rotator at the knee joint, which also—by being partly inserted into the posterior horn of the lateral meniscus—adjusts and protects this in the movement.

As rotation is possible with the knee in flexion, this allows for twisting to occur under the full load of the body; when this happens without good muscle control, the menisci (particularly the medial) become at risk.

In classical ballet, 'turn-out' is an important feature, essentially to give free range of lateral movement at the hips, where the whole of the movement should occur. Unfortunately, for far too many people the direction of the toes is the important feature, so that rotation at the knee is forced, gradually stretching the ligaments and producing an unstable knee joint; a common legacy of dancers trained to a poor teacher's concept (**Figures 219A and B**).

The femora mounted on either side of the pelvis, converge to the knee, which shows a degree of **angulation** between them and the parallel tibiae; an angulation greater in females due to the wider pelvis needed for parturition. Due to the greater angulation, where there is laxity of the medial ligaments and their supporting muscles, a degree of **knock-knee (genu valgum)** may occur in females (**Figure 220**). It may even be seen in overweight boys. The greater angulation of the knee, against the straight pull of the quadriceps muscles, is responsible for the common spontaneous lateral dislocation of the patella in females.

Examination of the knee joint begins with the free ranges of **flexion and extension**. **Rotation** can be tested with the knee at about 60° of flexion, holding and using the foot as a lever and measure; 30–40° should be possible in each direction. In extension none should be possible. Laxity of the **collateral ligaments** can be tested in extension with thigh muscles relaxed: hold the lower leg in one hand and with the other hand press the knee firmly from each side.

The **cruciate ligaments** create much of the internal stability of the joint and, in particular, prevent the femur from riding forwards on the tibial table, especially when walking down a slope. They should be taut in extension and also in full flexion, but a slight relaxation occurs, greatest at about 60°,

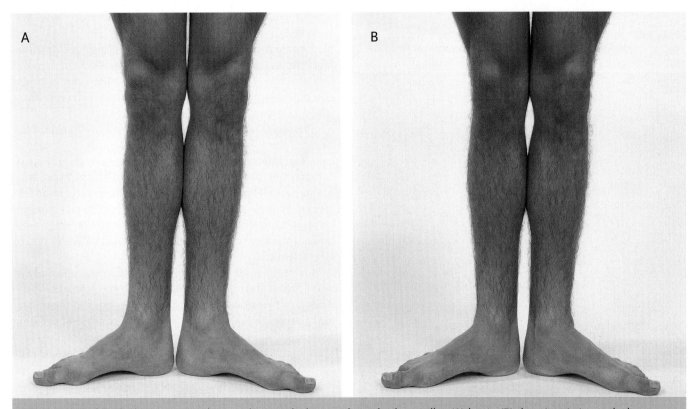

Figure 219A and B The legs are correctly 'turned out' at the hips as shown by the patellae (**A**) but in (**B**) there is twisting at the knee.

allowing rotation in the joint. Testing the ligaments is usually carried out in mid-flexion. The foot is fixed and the upper part of the leg is gripped, pressing the tibia backwards and forwards on the femur (**Figure 221**). With normal cruciate ligaments the movement should be no more than a few millimetres.

MUSCLES ACTING OVER THE HIP JOINT

Although most muscles acting over the hip joint run between the pelvis and femur, **psoas major**, one of the **two main flexors**, takes origin from the bodies and intervertebral discs of the upper lumbar vertebrae. Here they could readily increase lumbar lordosis, rather than raise the leg, unless the pelvis is firmly fixed on the trunk; this is a **prime function of the abdominal muscles**. Thus, flexion of the leg whilst lying supine is an excellent exercise for abdominal wall muscles. The other main flexor is **iliacus**, which runs from the inner aspect of the ilium to join psoas on its lateral side and, passing over the front of the hip joint, runs into the lesser trochanter.

Although the lesser trochanter is on the medial aspect of the femur, it is lateral to the axis-of-movement at the hip joint so that these muscles have an accessory function of **medial rotation**—a function often misunderstood. However, in fracture of the femoral neck the femur loses its connection with the hip joint, and the muscles then act on a free femoral shaft, inducing lateral rotation. A diagnostic sign of the fracture is a turned-out foot.

As both muscles lie deeply, examination depends on testing the power of hip flexion. Both are innervated by lumbar nerves, mainly L2 and L3.

Pectineus arises from the superior ramus of the pubis and runs down, medial to psoas, to be inserted below the lesser trochanter. It acts as a flexor-adductor at the hip joint, with some medial rotation. It lies deeply in the medial aspect of the femoral triangle of the groin, where it may be felt contracting on resisted flexion-adduction, just lateral to the tendon of adductor longus (**Figure 222**), though it is not easy to dissociate from the adductor. It is innervated by the femoral nerve (L2–L4), but may receive obturator nerve supply from the same roots.

The three adductor muscles form a powerful mass on the inner aspect of the thigh and are readily palpable on forced adduction.

Adductor longus is attached to the pubis, just below the pubic tubercle, by a thick tendon that is obvious even in an obese person when the leg is adducted against resistance, hence acting as a useful pointer to the tubercle (see page 96).

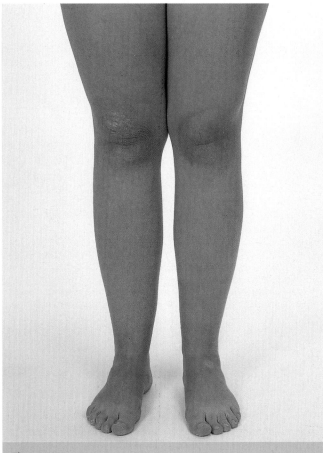

Figure 220

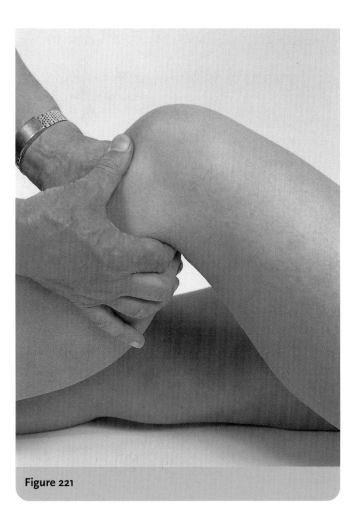

Figure 221

It also stands out when stretched in the abducted leg (**Figure 222**). Inserted into the linea aspera on the back of the femur, the muscle is a flexor-adductor with some medial rotation. It raises a ridge in the groin and, with that of sartorius laterally, makes a triangular hollow—the femoral triangle—with the inguinal ligament as its base (**Figure 222**). Within this triangle are the important vessels and nerves of the front of the thigh.

Adductor brevis lies immediately behind adductor longus but, being shorter and deeper, is not palpable from the surface.

Adductor magnus is a large muscle with a wide attachment to the inferior ramus of the pubis and to the medial aspect of the ischial tuberosity (alongside the hamstrings). It runs into the linea aspera and then along the medial supracondylar line to the adductor tubercle of the femur, to which it is attached by a thin tendon. It forms much of the thick mass of muscle on the medial side of the thigh, behind adductor longus. Below it is crossed by gracilis and sartorius, but its tendon is readily palpable in the anterior aspect of the hollow on the medial side of the thigh, above the medial epicondyle (see **Figure 228**, page 114). The anterior part of the muscle acts as a powerful adductor, while in adduction its lateral rotating function balances the medial rotation of adductor longus. The ischial portion acts with the hamstrings in hip extension.

All three adductors are innervated by the obturator nerve (L2–L4), with the hamstring part of adductor magnus receiving a branch from the sciatic nerve.

The adductors have an important role in giving a medial balance to the hip joint in locomotion, but in addition they act as emergency antigravity muscles. When a person slips, these muscles come into powerful contraction to prevent the collapse of the bipod of the legs. Thus, a very common sports injury is an adductor strain, particularly affecting the attachment of the adductor longus tendon to the pubis.

Gluteus medius and gluteus minimus are two large and powerful abductors at the hip joint, forming much of the bulk of the upper part of the buttock and running from the outer aspect of the ilium to the greater trochanter. Gluteus medius is the more superficial and overlies the deeper and more anteriorly placed minimus. If the leg is free to move, they act as abductors of the thigh on the pelvis, but their more important function is to support the trunk on the standing leg (**Figures 223 and 226**) and, by slightly raising the pelvis, to allow the other leg to swing free of the ground in walking or running. Gluteus minimus also has a medial-rotating role, which carries the pelvis forward on the supporting leg for the next step. Both muscles are supplied by the superior gluteal nerve (L4–L5 and S1). Testing for the muscles is by abduction of the thigh at the hip, but if the muscles or their nerve supply are lost, attempts to stand on the leg of the affected side will cause

1 Adductor longus	5 Femoral triangle
2 Pectineus	6 Position of inguinal
3 Iliopsoas	ligament
4 Sartorius	7 Inguinal fold

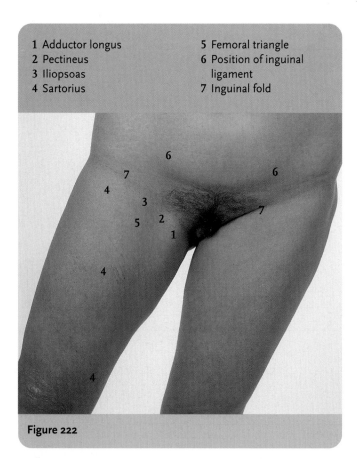

Figure 222

1 Gluteus maximus	6 Semimembranosus
2 Gluteus medius	(tendon)
3 Gluteus minimus	7 Biceps femoris (tendon)
4 Hamstrings group	8 Adductor magnus
5 Semitendinosus (tendon)	9 Iliac crest

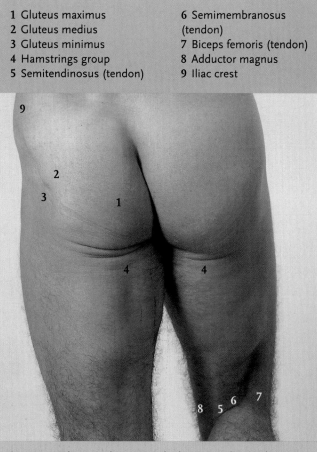

Figure 223 When one leg is raised, gluteus medius and minimus on the supporting side come into action to raise and support the pelvis, but gluteus maximus remains relaxed.

the pelvis to drop to the other side (**Figure 224**). The person will walk with a **Trendelenburg gait**, the pelvis dropping when on the supporting leg of the affected side—a walk also seen in congenital dislocation of the hip—though here it will be due to the head of the femur slipping up over the ilium rather than being held as normal in the acetabulum.

LATERAL ROTATORS

Deep in the gluteal region are a series of muscles, all of which are dynamic close postural supporters of the hip joint and lateral rotators. They are **obturator externus**, innervated by the obturator nerve (L2–L4); **obturator internus**, innervated by L5 and S1–S2; **pyriformis**, innervated by branches from S1–S2; **quadratus femoris**, innervated from L4–L5 and S1, and these supported by the small **gemelli**. They are collectively responsible for the power of lateral rotation at the hip joint alone. As such they are the vital prime moving control muscles in the 'turn-out' of classical ballet. It is also this excellent local control from the musculature around the joint that plays an important part after total hip replacement, when control of the joint system may be so rapidly restored.

MUSCLES ACTING OVER THE HIP AND KNEE JOINTS

Gluteus maximus is the superficial muscle of the lower part of the buttock and is the one responsible, with the overlying fat, for producing the rounded contour (**Figure 223**). It comes from the back of the ilium (close to the posterior superior iliac spine), the sacrum and the sacrotuberous and sacrospinous ligaments, to run downwards and laterally across the buttock. The deeper and lower fibres run into the **gluteal tuberosity** on the femur, but the greater proportion of the muscle goes to the **iliotibial tract**, a thick tendinous sheet running to the anterolateral aspect of the tibia. The total function of gluteus maximus is extension and lateral rotation at the hip joint, and extension at the knee—the function seen in the extended leg of a dancer performing an arabesque (see **figure 194**, page 95). It is important in standing up from a sitting position or in climbing steps, when its lateral-rotating function balances the medial rotation of glutei medius and minimus, acting to support the trunk on the leg (**Figure 226**). Its role over the knee is secondary to that of the quadriceps muscles, its pull through the iliotibial tract only coming into effective action when the knee is extended beyond 50–60° of flexion. The

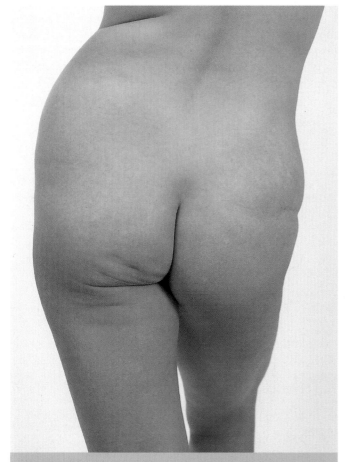

Figure 224 If standing with both feet on the ground all would appear normal, on raising the right leg the left abductor muscles fail to support the pelvis, which therefore drops.

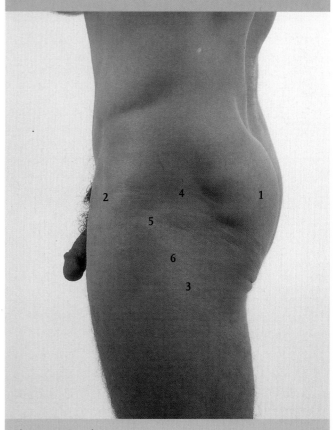

1 Gluteus maximus
2 Tensor fascia lata
3 Iliotibial tract
4 Gluteus medius
5 Gluteus minimus
6 Greater trochanter

Figure 225 Standing on toes.

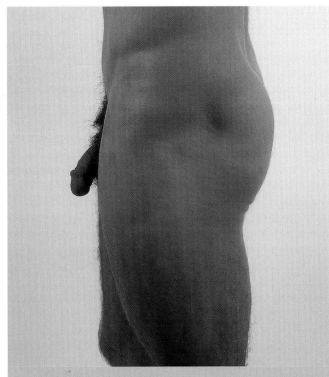

Figure 226 While remaining standing on the toes (see **Figure 225**) of the left leg, the right leg has been raised from the ground. Gluteus medius and minimus come into powerful contraction on this side to support the pelvis, thus producing a greater bulge above and between gluteus maximus tensor fascia lata.

most important function of the pull of the iliotibial tract is to produce firm compacted extension of the knee (**Figure 225**). The nerve supply is from the inferior gluteal nerve (L5 and S1–S2).

Tensor fasciae lata arises from the crest of the ilium, between the anterior superior spine and the tubercle (**Figures 225–227**). It joins the anterior aspect of the iliotibial tract, acting as a flexor at the hip and an extensor of the knee. Although normally a subsidiary flexor at the hip, it can hypertrophy and take on the role where iliopsoas is lost. Its most important function is to produce an anterior postural balance to gluteus maximus in hip control, while together giving postural control over the knee (**Figure 225**). Loss of the muscle produces a degree of instability, particularly evident in walking. It is supplied by the superior gluteal nerve (L4–L5 and S1).

Sartorius is a long strap-like muscle that runs from the anterior superior iliac spine region, obliquely downwards and medially across the front of the thigh, to the medial side of the upper part of the tibia (**Figures 227 and 228**). Sartorius is a flexor-abductor and lateral rotator at the hip, and a flexor and medial rotator at the knee. It influences the contours of the thigh anteriorly, where it forms the lateral margin of the femoral triangle (see **Figure 222**). It is supplied by branches of the femoral nerve, one of which runs through the muscle and becomes the intermediate cutaneous nerve of the thigh.

Gracilis runs subcutaneously down the medial aspect of the thigh from the pubis to the medial side of the tibia, between sartorius and semitendinosus. It is a weak adductor at the hip and an accessory flexor at the knee with medial

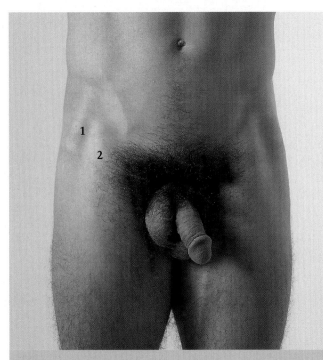

Figure 227 The bulges created by tensor fascia latae (1) and sartorius (2) can be seen; the latter running down from the anterior superior immediately behind.

1 Sartorius
2 Gracilis
3 Semitendinosus and semimembranosus
4 Vastus medialis
5 Adductor magnus tendon inserted into medial femoral epicondyle
6 Medial femoral condyle
7 Patella
8 Tibial condyle
9 Medial ligament of knee joint
10 Insertions of sartorius, gracilis and semitendinosus into tibia

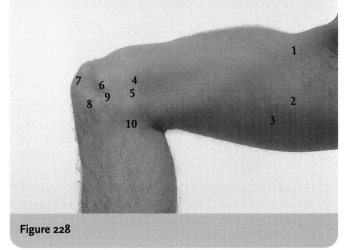

Figure 228

rotation in flexion. With sartorius and semitendinosus, it forms a thick muscle mass running down the inner aspect of the thigh, giving medial support to the medial ligament of the knee joint and supporting its angulation (**Figure 228**). Gracilis is supplied by the obturator nerve (L2–L4).

HAMSTRING MUSCLES

These are three muscles, all arising from the ischial tuberosity and running down the back of the thigh, where they form the main bulk.

Semitendinosus runs into a long tendon which is inserted into the medial side of the tibia, behind sartorius and gracilis, where, in addition to its hamstring function, it assists in supporting the medial side of the knee joint.

Semimembranosus is inserted into the posteromedial aspect of the tibia.

Biceps femoris has one head from the ischial tuberosity and another from the back of the femur. The two bellies combine in the lower part of the thigh to form a tendon that is attached to the head of the fibula, with the lateral collateral ligament of the knee joint (see **Figure 217** , page 109 and **Figure 229**).

The components of the hamstrings, by running to each side of the lower thigh, produce the hollow behind the knee, containing fat and the main vessels and nerves: the **popliteal fossa (Figure 229)**.

The nerve supply comes from the sciatic nerve: for semi-membranosus and semitendinosus, from L4–L5 and S1; for the long head of biceps, from the medial component, S1–S3; for the short head of biceps, from the lateral component (common peroneal), L5 and S1.

The hamstrings act as powerful axial extensors at the hip joint and flexors at the knee (the short head of biceps acting there alone). Because they run to the medial and lateral sides at the knee, they also give vital collateral support to this vulnerable joint. The hamstrings cannot act over the full range of both joints at once; they show active and passive insufficiency. Because of limitation of movement by the hamstrings, it is important to measure ranges of hip flexion with the knee bent. Full flexion at the hip joint with the knee straight may also pull on the sciatic nerve. If inflamed or under mechanical stress, as in lumbar disc lesions, pain may be induced, so being particularly useful as a test.

MUSCLES ACTING OVER THE KNEE JOINT

The **quadriceps muscles** form the mass on the front of the thigh. They are the main extensors and supporters of the knee joint. The patella acts as a sesamoid bone in the central tendon, so lifting the direction of pull to give better leverage for knee extension (**Figure 230**).

Rectus femoris crosses close to the hip joint, but its activ-

1 Iliotibial tract	5 Popliteal fossa
2 Biceps femoris	6 Head of fibula
3 Semimembranosus	
4 Lateral head of gastrocnemius	

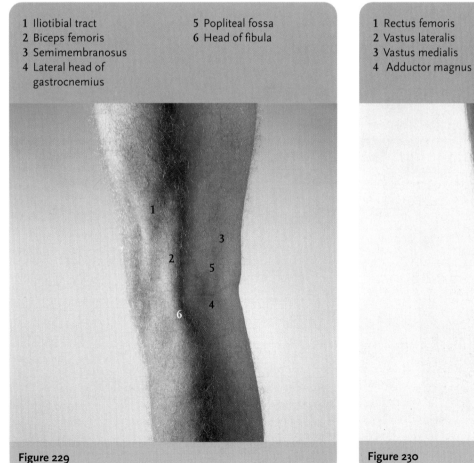

Figure 229

1 Rectus femoris	5 Iliotibial tract
2 Vastus lateralis	6 Patella
3 Vastus medialis	7 Patellar ligament
4 Adductor magnus	8 Tibial tuberosity

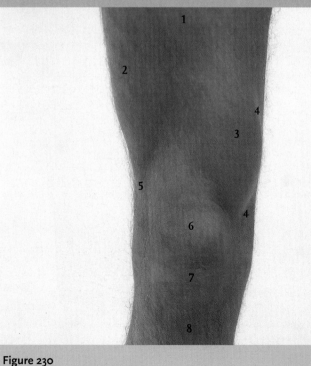

Figure 230

Chapter 10 The legs

ity is primarily to support the joint and limit extension. The muscle belly runs superficially down the thigh to the patella, where, in a muscular person, it is easily seen contracting in firm extension of the knee (**Figure 230**).

Vastus intermedius is a broad mass of muscle covering the front and sides of the femur, deep to rectus femoris.

Vastus lateralis arises from the greater trochanter and along the linea aspera, forming a muscle mass that overlies the lateral aspect of vastus intermedius.

Vastus medialis has its origins much farther down the thigh than the other muscles (**Figures 230 and 231**).

The central components of the quadriceps, rectus and much of vastus intermedius run into the patella and through this, via the ligamentum patellae, to the lower part of the tibial tubercle, giving prime extensor power. Laterally an aponeurotic sheet is formed above the level of the patella and this runs over the lateral side of the joint. On the medial side vastus medialis runs almost horizontally into the medial side of the patella and also forms an aponeurosis over the medial side of the joint to the tibia.

In addition to the important extensor role of the quadriceps and their widely embracing support for the front of this vulnerable joint, the vastus medialis also exerts a medial pull on the patella, controlling its possible lateral dislocation (**Figure 231**), as the other quadriceps pull straight across the angle of the knee joint. These muscles are responsible for much of the stability of the knee, and any weakness commonly leads to synovitis of the joint, even on mild exercise such as walking. Consequently, anyone spending more than 1 or 2 days in bed should maintain quadriceps exercises unless otherwise contraindicated. Nerve supply comes from the femoral nerve (L2–L4).

Due to the range of movement of the patella in flexion and extension, a large synovial extension, the **deep suprapatellar bursa**, runs up from the joint beneath the quadriceps muscles, to about three fingers' breadth above the patella. In marked levels of synovitis of the knee, the swelling is very obvious (water on the knee), but where there is less, a method of testing is the so-called **patellar tap**. A hand is placed around the thigh, immediately above the patella, and pressed down on the suprapatellar bursa, so that any fluid there is pushed down beneath the patella. The patella is then pushed against the femur and will be felt to tap against it if fluid separates them.

A

B

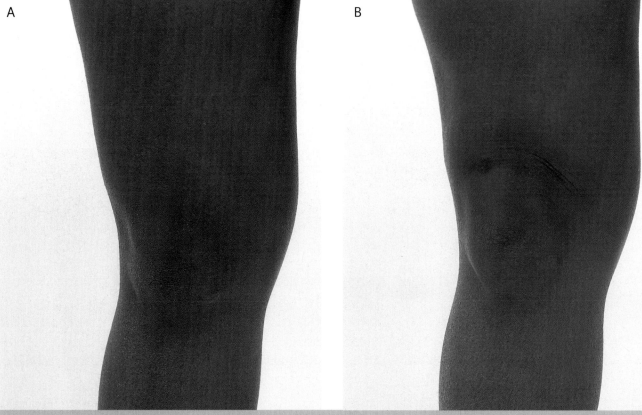

Figure 231A and B In a female the muscular pattern may be less obvious, owing to a greater amount of subcutaneous fat (**A**). On contraction of the quadriceps the patella is pulled up with good medial control from vastus medialis, in spite of the angulation of the knee (**B**).

BONY FEATURES OF THE ANKLE AND FOOT

The subcutaneous surface and sharp anterior border of the **tibia** (the shin) run down the whole length of the leg, from the tibial tubercle to the ankle. Here the **medial malleolus** projects to the medial side of the talus, the tarsal bone with which the tibia articulates (**Figure 233**). Laterally the **head of the fibula** is readily palpable below the knee but the shaft is overlaid by muscles, becoming subcutaneous again in its lowest quarter, continuing down to the lateral side of the talus as the **lateral malleolus (Figure 232)**. The lateral malleolus is triangular and projects farther down the articular surface of the talus than does the medial malleolus. (In lateral radiographs the differences in length and shape of the two malleoli are important in differentiating them.) Behind the malleoli are hollows and behind them the **tendo calcaneus (Achillis)** runs into the prominent projection of the **calcaneum** at the heel.

Below the lateral malleolus and slightly anterior to its tip, the **peroneal tubercle** can be felt (**Figure 232**). In front of the lateral malleolus, the **talus** is palpable for a short distance before sinking at its neck. If the foot is inverted, the **head of the talus** forms a projection on the supralateral aspect of the foot, 3–4 cm in front of the lateral malleolus; in midposition it is masked by the subjacent extensor digitorum brevis muscle. Along the lateral side of a slim foot the **distal end of the calcaneum** may be felt, but then the hollow over the **cuboid** leads to the next prominence, the base of the **fifth metatarsal**.

On the medial side it may be possible to feel a little of the talus just below the medial malleolus, particularly if the foot is everted in plantar flexion, with the shelf of the **sustentaculum tali** below. Underneath that is a hollow of the calcaneum and then the prominence of the heel with its firm padding. More anteriorly the **tubercle of the navicula** forms a low bony prominence and more distally the **medial cuneiform**, while the base of the **first metatarsal** may be palpable (**Figure 233**).

On the dorsum **the base of the first metatarsal** forms a large knob in some people, which can often lead to uncomfortable pressure from shoes. The shafts of the **metatarsals** should be palpable through the extensor tendons, while the first and fifth are prominent on the border of the foot, through to their heads. The **head of the first metatarsal** may project to a considerable extent, overlaid by a bursa—another possible pressure zone in shoes. This may become greater in hallux valgus, producing a bunion.

On the sole of the foot the **heads of the metatarsals** are overlaid by a thick pad of fibro-fatty material, with sesamoid bones in the tendons of the first and sometimes other toes. This is the normal load-bearing area of the forefoot, together with the heel and the lateral border (**Figure 234**). The **medial side of the sole of the foot should show a variable level of arching**. Contact between the pads of the toes and the ground will depend upon their mobility and normality of position.

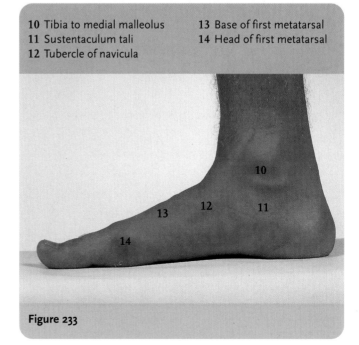

1 Fibula to lateral malleolus	5 Cuboid
2 Peroneal tubercle	6 Base of fifth metatarsal
3 Talus (distal end)	7 Peroneal tendons
4 Extensor digitorum brevis muscle	8 Tendo calcaneus
	9 Calcaneum

Figure 232

10 Tibia to medial malleolus	13 Base of first metatarsal
11 Sustentaculum tali	14 Head of first metatarsal
12 Tubercle of navicula	

Figure 233

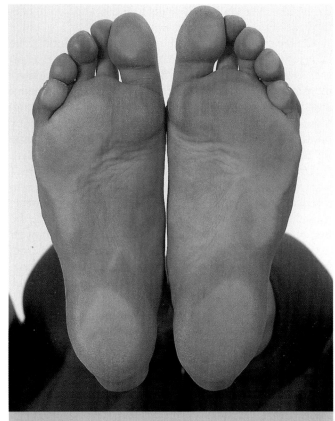

Figure 234 Load bearing areas of normal feet in stance as in Figure 236A.

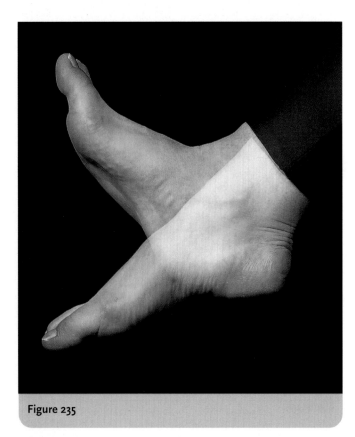

Figure 235

MOVEMENTS OF THE ANKLE AND FOOT

The ankle joint is a uni-axial joint, permitting only flexion and extension (plantar- and dorsiflexion) of the foot. From the normal standing position, with the foot at right angles to the leg, it should be capable of 30–40° of dorsiflexion and around 60° of plantar-flexion (**Figure 235**). However, this varies enormously with types and utilisation of the feet. People who have worn high-heeled shoes constantly, without walking at normal foot level, may not be able to reach 90° of angulation and may not be able to put the heel to the ground without pain in the shortened calf muscles. The same problem may affect patients who have been nursed, for even a short time, with the feet held in plantar-flexion by bedcovers, unless the calf muscles are regularly stretched.

In a normal standing position and in dorsiflexion, the talus fits closely between the two malleoli, when the foot can be considered to be in a stable close-packed position at the ankle joint. However, the malleolar surfaces of the talus are narrower posteriorly, allowing the talus to be free to rock between the malleoli in plantar-flexion. Hence, when standing on the toes (or in high-heeled shoes) the **ankle loses its lateral stability** unless firmly supported by the long muscles, whose tendons run over each side and into the foot.

From the ankle the dynamic axis of the foot runs through to the medial three toes. The lateral side is much more static, designed to take load when standing (together with the padded metatarsal heads and the heel). Medially the arch running from the calcaneum to the medial three metatarsal heads forms a cantilever-spring-like mechanism when landing, as from a jump, and a dynamically sprung lever when driving off or jumping, to allow a free-flowing movement through the foot. The importance lies in the **muscle-controlled dynamic mobility of the arch system** rather than the arch itself (**Figure 236**).

As the medial part of the foot to the inner three toes forms the dynamic component, this is where rotatory movement occurs within the foot, to allow it to adjust to variable surfaces. The lateral aspect of the foot follows around this medial axis. The head of the talus fits in a ball-and-socket joint with the navicular, permitting flexion, extension, inversion and eversion. The navicula has a similar but shallower joint system with the three cuneiform bones but thereafter, rotation is blocked by the base of the second metatarsal being held between the distal parts of the medial and lateral cuneiform bones. Movement thence is flexion and extension, though some abduction and adduction should be possible at the metatarsophalangeal joints. The lateral part of the foot largely follows round, initiated by a twisting movement between talus and calcaneum. The foot is capable of a considerable range of inversion but much less eversion (**Figure 237**).

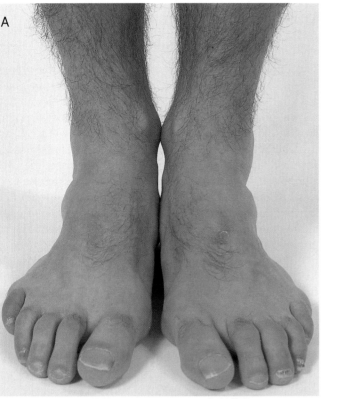

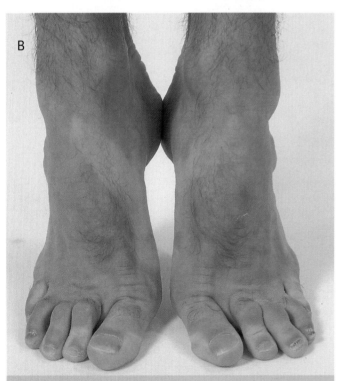

Figure 236A and B The feet of a highly trained dancer may appear relatively flat when at rest (**A**). When standing on toes, however, the medial arch develops to a remarkable extent (**B**). Note how the three medial metatarsals and toes take most of the load and would be responsible for the drive if jumping or to produce a sprung system on landing. It is easy to see by the squeezing out of the blood from the toes how much load these are being subjected to. An efficient foot makes considerable use of the power of the toes.

MUSCLES ACTING OVER THE KNEE AND ANKLE

Gastrocnemius runs both over the knee and, combined with soleus, over the ankle joint. It forms the main bulge of the upper calf, arising by two heads, one from each of the supracondylar regions of the femur and lying inside the tendons of the hamstrings. The two heads join below, so forming, with the hamstrings, the diamond-shaped popliteal fossa. Both of these systems act as flexors at the knee and, by their bilateral attachments, not only give lateral support to the joint but can also rotate the flexed knee.

The two bellies of gastrocnemius join below the knee, overlying and being attached to a tendinous sheet on the upper part of soleus, the two muscles then running down to form the common tendo calcaneus (Achillis). Gastrocnemius is a prime flexor at the knee and supports soleus as an extensor at the ankle joint. **Soleus** arises from the back of the tibia and from a fibrous arch stretching over the popliteal vessels and tibial nerve, to the fibula. The soleal fibres can be seen bulging to each side of gastrocnemius, when both are in action (**Figure 238**). The soleus/gastrocnemius complex is the power

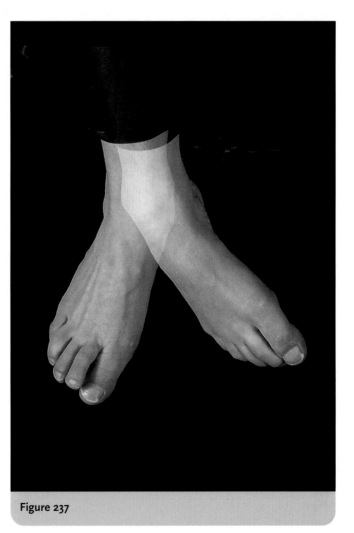

Figure 237

plantar-flexor at the ankle joint (**Figure 240**) and is also responsible for preventing the body from falling forwards when standing, so maintaining it in balance over the feet.

Plantaris is a very small muscle, but its long tendon can be of great value as a graft and so it is important to be able to find it easily. It can be taken through a small incision two fingers' breadth behind the medial malleolus and just in front of the tendo calcaneus. The whole tendon can then be harvested using a stripper.

All three muscles are supplied by the tibial nerve, S1–S2.

MUSCLES ACTING OVER THE ANKLE AND FOOT

The long muscles acting over the ankle run in three groups. Tibialis anterior and extensors hallucis and digitorum longus pass in front; tibialis posterior and flexors hallucis and digitorum longus run behind the medial malleolus; peroneus longus and brevis pass behind the lateral malleolus.

Tibialis anterior has a large muscle belly, arising from and running superficially alongside the tibia. It crosses the ankle a little lateral to the medial malleolus, where it raises a thick ridge when the muscle acts in dorsiflexion and inversion of the foot (**Figure 239**). It has the important function of maintaining normal dorsiflexion of the foot when raised from the ground, and loss of the muscle, usually its nerve supply, leads to the very disabling condition of foot drop when walking. Its tendon runs into the medial cuneiform and the base of the first metatarsal. It is innervated by the deep peroneal nerve (anterior tibial)—L4–L5.

Extensor hallucis longus arises deep to extensor digitorum longus, from the middle third of the fibula and the interosseous membrane. Its tendon becomes superficial in

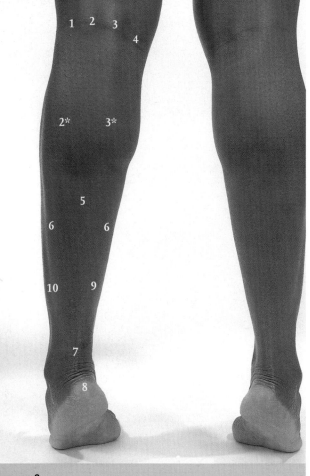

1 Biceps femoris tendon
2 Lateral head
2* Lateral belly of gastrocnemius } of gastro
3 Medial head of gastrocnemius
3* Medial belly of gastrocnemius } of gastro
4 Semimembranosus
5 Combined tendon of gastrocnemius and soleus, whose muscle belly is attached to its deep-set aspect (6)
7 Tendo calcaneus (Achillis)
8 Calcaneum
9 Flexor digitorum longus
10 Peroneus longus and brevis

Figure 238

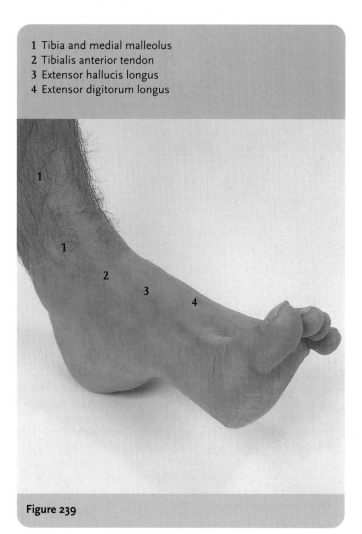

1 Tibia and medial malleolus
2 Tibialis anterior tendon
3 Extensor hallucis longus
4 Extensor digitorum longus

Figure 239

the approach to the ankle, just lateral to tibialis anterior, and becomes obvious on the dorsum of the foot on forced extension of the big toe (**Figure 239**). (Nerve supply: deep peroneal nerve, L5 and S1.)

Extensor digitorum longus arises from the upper ²/₃ of the fibula and immediately lateral to tibialis anterior. It can be felt in digital extension and most effectively in eversion, when tibialis anterior is relaxed (**Figure 241**). It divides into four tendons that pass under the extensor retinaculum, lateral to extensor hallucis longus, with the vessels and nerve between them. (Nerve supply: deep peroneal, L5 and S1.)

Peroneus tertius arises below extensor digitorum longus and runs down lateral to it, to be inserted into the base of the fifth metatarsal. Although often described as part of extensor digitorum longus, with the same nerve supply, it is an important extensor-evertor of the foot (**Figure 241**).

Tibialis posterior arises deep to soleus, appearing at the ankle, medial to the tendo calcaneus and crossing close behind the medial malleolus, where the tendon can be felt moving in firm or resisted inversion and plantar-flexion (**Figure 240**). It is inserted into the navicula, with slips to the other tarsal bones except the talus. (Nerve supply: tibial nerve, L4–L5.)

Flexor digitorum longus also arises from the tibia, beneath soleus and runs down across the ankle, immediately behind tibialis posterior as the long flexor to the toes (**Figure 240**). It is supplied by the tibial nerve, L5 and S1.

1 Tibia
2 Gastrocnemius (medial)
3 Soleus
4 Tendo calcaneus
5 Medial malleolus
6 Tendon of tibialis posterior
7 Tendon of flexor digitorum longus
8 Flexor accessorius
9 Abductor hallucis
10 Tendon of tibialis anterior

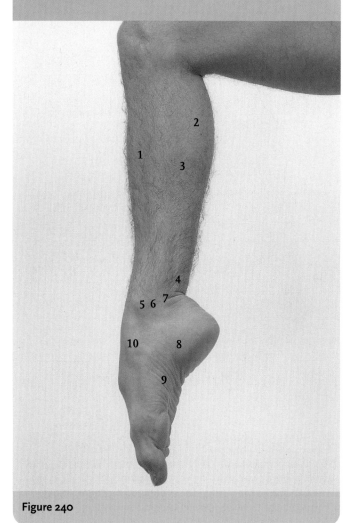

Figure 240

1   Fibula
1*   Lateral malleolus
2   Tendon of peroneus longus overlying belly of peroneus brevis
2*   Tendon of peroneus longus
2** Tendon of peroneus brevis
3   Extensor digitorum brevis
4   Tubercle of fifth metatarsal
5   Abductor digiti minimi
6   Tendon of peroneus tertius
7   Tendons of extensor digitorum longus
8   Tendon of extensor hallucis

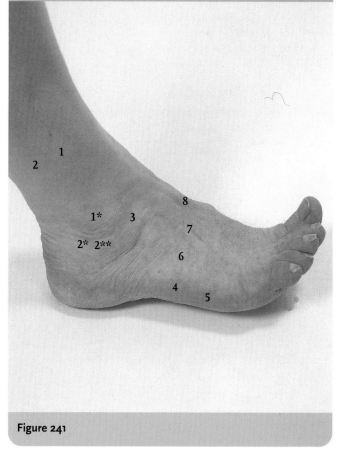

Figure 241

Flexor hallucis longus also arises deep to soleus, from the fibula, and runs down deep to the tendo calcaneus and lateral to flexor digitorum longus, the tendon of which it crosses in the sole of the foot, to reach the great toe as its long flexor. (Nerve supply: tibial nerve, L5 and S1–S3.)

Peroneus longus arises from the upper $^2/_3$ of the fibula and the adjoining lateral tibial condyle and runs down behind the lateral malleolus and then below the peroneal tubercle and across the sole of the foot (**Figures 241 and 242**).

Peroneus brevis arises below peroneus longus and also runs behind the lateral malleolus but then above the peroneal tubercle, to the base of the fifth metatarsal.

Both peroneal muscles are evertors of the foot and flexors, and are supplied by the superficial peroneal nerve, L5 and S1–S2.

Short muscles of the foot are most important for a functionally effective foot, although the long muscles give the main power. The great toe has a short abductor, a flexor and an adductor, the last playing a major part in maintaining the inter-nal strength across the foot. The **abductor** runs along the medial border of the foot and, in most people, merely gives a medial balance to the toe. In people who use their feet effectively, such as dancers (particularly classical-ballet dancers who have to dance 'on point'), the muscle is vitally important. In many feet, particularly women's, the muscle fails, leading to hallux valgus (and the development of a bunion). Those with an **early** tendency to this can often prevent further deterioration, and even gain improvement, by reactivating the abductor function of the muscle (**Figure 243**).

The other toes have two short flexors. **Flexor digitorum brevis** has the same insertion characters as flexor digitorum superficialis in the hand. **Flexor digitorum accessorius** arises from the hollow on the medial side of the calcaneum (**Figure 228**), below the medial malleolus, where it can be felt contracting in digital flexion. Its tendons join those of flexor digitorum longus and it has the function of maintaining digital flexion when the long muscle has to relax, as in dorsiflexion at the ankle.

1   Lower end of fibula
1* Lateral malleolus
2   Peroneus longus muscle (2* tendon)
3   Peroneus brevis muscle (3* tendon)
4   Superior peroneal retinaculum
5   Lateral belly of gastrocnemius
6   Soleus
7   Tendo calcaneus
7* Position of bursa between tendon and calcaneum
8   Extensor digitorum brevis
9   Peroneus tertius muscle (9* tendon)
10 Tuberosity of fifth metatarsal
11 Abductor digiti minimi

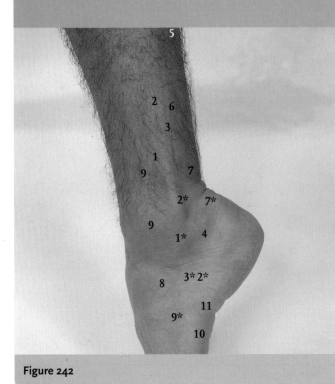

Figure 242

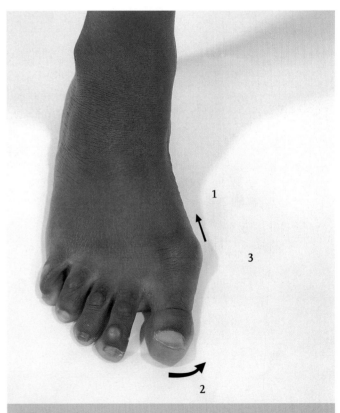

Figure 243 At rest the great toe lay alongside the other toes. Abductor pollicis brevis (**1**) has been activated, pulling the great toe to a more normal position (**2**), so reducing the angle at the metatarsophalangeal joint, where a bunion might eventually form (**3**) if the toe were allowed to continue 'drifting'.

The long extensors also have short-muscle support in **extensors hallucis and digitorum brevis**, which arise mainly from the upper surface of the calcaneum (**Figure 241**). Although these muscles are vital in people with active feet, such as dancers, they are of relatively little daily importance in the general population and can, therefore, provide valuable tendon grafts in such.

The interossei are important in the foot, as they are in the hand. The long and short flexors operate on the interphalangeal joints and, acting alone, will produce clawing, as seen so often in feet. However, the interossei are also flexors at the metatarsophalangeal joints and here, with the lumbricals, balance with the extensors to prevent clawing. They thus complete the full control of the foot, from the ankle through the midtarsal joints to the toes. The need to maintain the strength of the 'short muscles of the foot' is well known enough and exercises are often prescribed to achieve this. A totally unacceptable one, so often advised, is to pick up a pencil by the toes, which only aggravates clawing. Flexion must be concentrated on the metatarsophalangeal joints for effective foot function.

The muscles are supplied by the medial and lateral plantar nerves.

RETINACULA AND SYNOVIAL SHEATHS OF THE FOOT

The three groups of tendons passing the ankle are all controlled by retinacula, made of thickenings in the deep fascia, and are lubricated by synovial sheaths. Their positions are shown in **Figures 244**.

The **synovial sheaths** are individual for each tendon except for the extensor digitorum longus and peroneus tertius, which is combined. The other two peroneal tendons have their sheaths joined proximally.

As in the hand, the flexor tendons to the toes have synovial sheaths through the fibrous flexor sheaths to each toe.

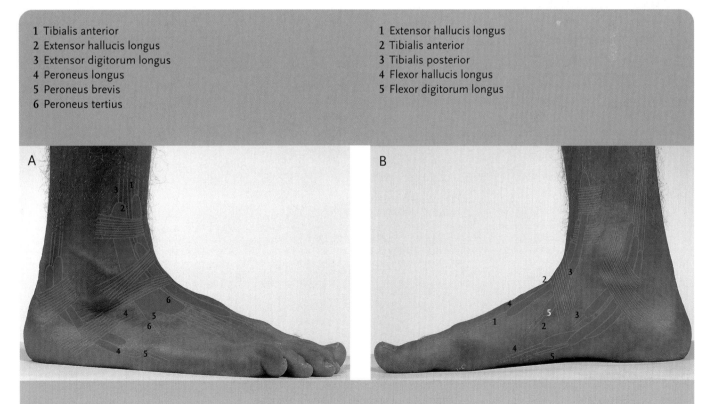

1 Tibialis anterior
2 Extensor hallucis longus
3 Extensor digitorum longus
4 Peroneus longus
5 Peroneus brevis
6 Peroneus tertius

1 Extensor hallucis longus
2 Tibialis anterior
3 Tibialis posterior
4 Flexor hallucis longus
5 Flexor digitorum longus

Figure 244A and B Projection of the synovial sheaths (blue) around the tendons passing across the ankle joint and beneath the retinacula (green).

THE NERVES OF THE LEGS

In the arm the segmental sensory innervation of the skin follows a relatively simple pattern. In the leg the simplicity has been disorganised by embryonic rotation, to bring the foot to the ground. Therefore, the posterior divisional nerves supply the front of the thigh and leg, while the anterior division supplies the medial side of the thigh, the back of the leg and the sole of the foot (**Figures 245–248**).

The **genitofemoral nerve** (L1–L2) runs down over the psoas muscle to give two branches. The **genital branch** passes through the external inguinal ring to supply the cremaster muscle and skin of the scrotum and adjacent thigh. The **femoral branch** runs with the external iliac and femoral arteries to supply an area of skin below the inguinal crease. The **cremasteric reflex** is a useful test of the upper lumbar spinal segments in a male.

The **lateral cutaneous nerve of the thigh** (L2–L3) enters the leg, under the extreme lateral end of the inguinal ligament, before piercing the deep fascia. It divides into two branches: the **anterior** supplies skin over the anterolateral aspect of the thigh and joins in the patellar plexus, while the **posterior** runs through the fascia lata to supply the lateral aspect of the leg from the greater trochanter to the lower thigh.

The nerve can be **blocked** in the region of the origin of sartorius to give adequate anaesthesia to the lateral aspect of the thigh. **Compression** of the nerve often occurs in its passage through the inguinal ligament and fascia, giving paraesthesia,

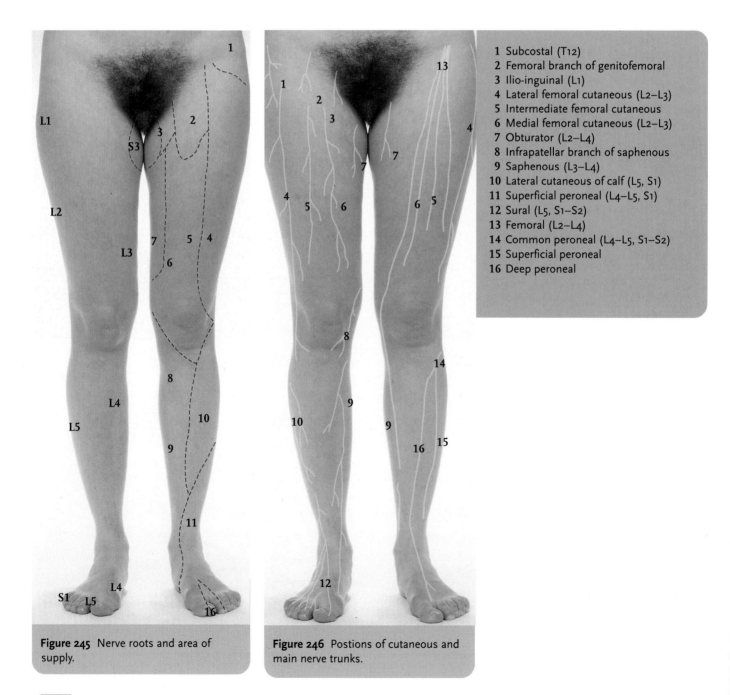

1 Subcostal (T12)
2 Femoral branch of genitofemoral
3 Ilio-inguinal (L1)
4 Lateral femoral cutaneous (L2–L3)
5 Intermediate femoral cutaneous
6 Medial femoral cutaneous (L2–L3)
7 Obturator (L2–L4)
8 Infrapatellar branch of saphenous
9 Saphenous (L3–L4)
10 Lateral cutaneous of calf (L5, S1)
11 Superficial peroneal (L4–L5, S1)
12 Sural (L5, S1–S2)
13 Femoral (L2–L4)
14 Common peroneal (L4–L5, S1–S2)
15 Superficial peroneal
16 Deep peroneal

Figure 245 Nerve roots and area of supply.

Figure 246 Postions of cutaneous and main nerve trunks.

particularly a burning sensation, and numbness over the area of supply (meralgia paraesthetica). This can be relieved surgically by local freeing of the nerve.

The femoral nerve (L2–L4, posterior division) runs under the inguinal ligament, a finger-breadth lateral to the femoral artery, the mid-inguinal point (see page 96), where the artery should be palpable. It gives **motor supply** to the quadriceps group of muscles, sartorius and usually pectineus.

The **cutaneous branches to the thigh** are the intermediate and medial cutaneous nerves. The **intermediate cutaneous nerve(s)** supplies the front of the thigh down to the knee (often arising as or with a branch to sartorius), while the **medial cutaneous nerve** pierces the deep fascia a little lower, to supply the medial side of the lower thigh and, by a **posterior branch**, the medial side of the leg below the knee. The **saphenous nerve**

is the largest of the sensory branches and follows the long saphenous vein down the leg and behind the medial condyle of the femur, to supply skin on the medial side of the leg, ankle and foot.

Loss of the femoral nerve is unusual, but if it occurs the loss of the quadriceps' control of the knee is serious. There would be sensory loss on the front of the thigh, but below the knee there is usually adequate overlap.

The **knee jerk** is a spinal stretch-reflex through the femoral nerve (L2–L4). With the knees bent and muscle relaxed, each patellar tendon is firmly tapped, thereby stretching the quadriceps. The normal response is a small kick.

The obturator nerve (L2–4, anterior division) passes as two branches through the obturator foramen, to supply the adductor muscles, and gives cutaneous supply to the medial side of

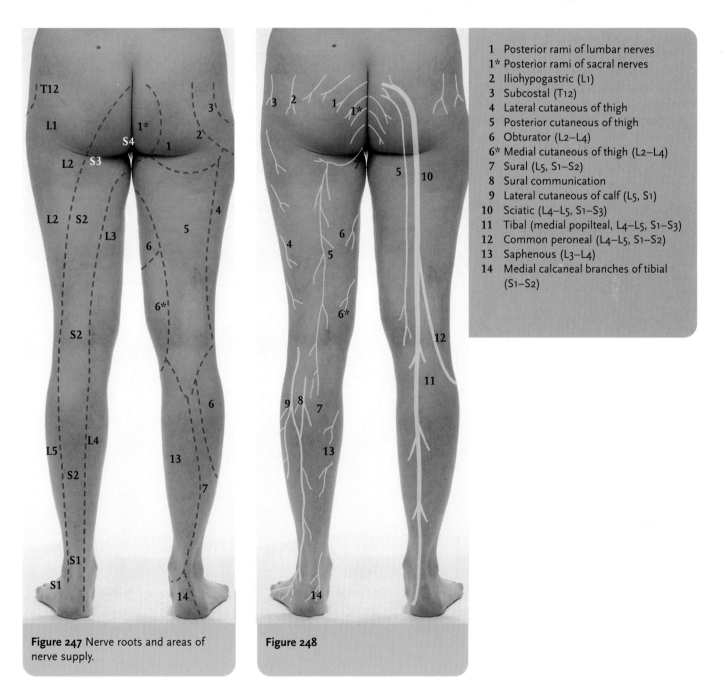

1   Posterior rami of lumbar nerves
1* Posterior rami of sacral nerves
2   Iliohypogastric (L1)
3   Subcostal (T12)
4   Lateral cutaneous of thigh
5   Posterior cutaneous of thigh
6   Obturator (L2–L4)
6* Medial cutaneous of thigh (L2–L4)
7   Sural (L5, S1–S2)
8   Sural communication
9   Lateral cutaneous of calf (L5, S1)
10 Sciatic (L4–L5, S1–S3)
11 Tibal (medial popilteal, L4–L5, S1–S3)
12 Common peroneal (L4–L5, S1–S2)
13 Saphenous (L3–L4)
14 Medial calcaneal branches of tibial (S1–S2)

Figure 247 Nerve roots and areas of nerve supply.

Figure 248

the upper thigh. The nerve gives sensory supply to both the hip and knee joints. As a result, **pathology in the hip joint commonly gives pain in the knee.**

The **sacral plexus** (L4–L5 and S1–S3) supplies the major part of the leg, other than the above. Branches are to quadratus femoris (L4–L5 and S1), obturator internus (L5 and S1–S2), pyriformis (S1–S2), the superior gluteal nerve (L4–L5 and S1) and the inferior gluteal nerve (L5 and S1–S2) have been noted with the muscles of supply. **S4 gives vital innervation to the pelvic diaphragm, including the anal sphincter.** The major components to the leg are the sciatic nerve and the sensory **posterior cutaneous nerve** to the back of the lower buttock, the perineum and the thigh, as far as the knee.

The **sciatic nerve** (L4–L5 and S1–S3) leaves the pelvis through the greater sciatic foramen to enter the gluteal region, about midway between the posterior superior iliac spine and the ischial tuberosity, and then curves downwards to pass just medial to midway between the ischial tuberosity and greater trochanter (**Figure 249**).

It is made up of medial and lateral components that (usually) later divide into the **tibial (medial popliteal) nerve**, from the anterior divisions of all roots, and the **common peroneal (lateral popliteal) nerve**, from the posterior divisions of all except S3.

The **common peroneal part** lies close to the acetabulum, behind the hip joint (**Figure 249**), where it may be damaged in operations on the joint or in such injuries as posterior fracture dislocation, resulting in foot drop.

Leaving the cover of gluteus maximus the sciatic nerve lies close beneath the deep fascia, where it is **vulnerable to injury**, but then runs deep again under biceps femoris. In the thigh it supplies all the hamstring muscles including the ischial component of adductor magnus.

The **tibial (medial popliteal) nerve** then continues through the centre of the popliteal fossa (**Figure 250**), supplying gastrocnemius, soleus, tibialis posterior, flexor hallucis longus and flexor digitorum longus, before entering the foot behind the medial malleolus. Here it is tucked in under the medial side of the tendo calcaneus and can be **palpated by pressure** over the calcaneum, just medial to the insertion of the tendon. It is readily available here for **local nerve block**. It then runs into the sole of the foot, where it divides into **medial and lateral plantar nerves**. These supply the short muscles of the foot: the medial gives cutaneous sensory supply to the medial part of the foot and $3\frac{1}{2}$ toes, while the lateral supplies the lateral side of the foot.

In the popliteal region the tibial nerve gives off **the sural nerve (Figure 250)**, which runs down the back of the leg, in

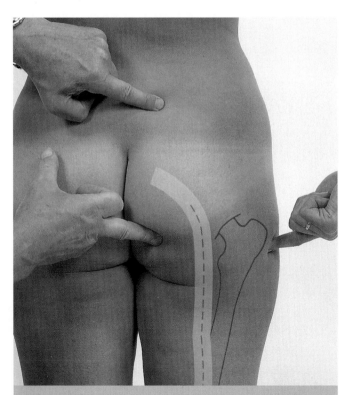

Figure 249 The fingers point to the posterior superior iliac spine, the ischial tuberosity and the greater trochanter. The positions of the femur and hip joint, lying anterior to the nerve, are indicated, as also is the possible division of the sciatic nerve into medial and lateral components.

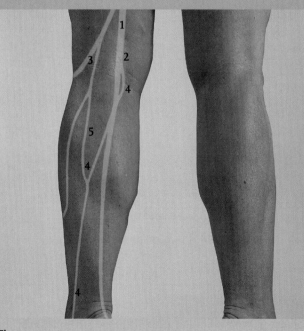

1 Sciatic nerve
2 Tibial (medial popliteal) nerve
3 Common peroneal (lateral popliteal) nerve
4 Sural nerve
5 Tibial nerve running behind medial malleolus (the tibial nerve divides below the medial malleolus into the lateral

Figure 250

company with the short saphenous vein, to supply (with the **sural communicating nerve** from the common peroneal nerve) the skin of the lower part of the calf and the lateral side of the foot and little toe. It runs into the foot behind the lateral malleolus.

The **common peroneal (lateral popliteal) nerve** runs along the medial side of the tendon of biceps and then winds forwards **around the neck of the fibula**, before entering peroneus longus, where it divides into **deep and superficial peroneal nerves**. The **deep peroneal nerve** supplies the four extensor muscles and then continues over the front of the ankle, between the tendons of extensors hallucis and digitorum longus, into the dorsum of the foot, with the dorsalis pedis artery, to supply the adjoining surfaces of the great and second toes. The **superficial peroneal (musculocutaneous) nerve** supplies the peroneal muscles, before going anterior to the lateral malleolus to supply most of the dorsum of the foot. The **lateral cutaneous nerve of the calf** leaves the common peroneal nerve in the popliteal fossa to supply the lateral aspect of the calf.

The **common peroneal nerve** is readily **palpable by pressure over the neck of the fibula (Figure 251)**. Here it is very **vulnerable to external trauma**, such as from the bumper of a car and, too often, from pressure from plaster casts etc. It is also readily accessible here for **electrical stimulation or local anaesthetic block**. Damage to the nerve here, or to the lateral component of the sciatic nerve near the hip joint, leads to foot drop, due to loss of the extensor muscles. The foot drops

and trails while being carried forwards when walking, with the need to throw the foot forwards by quick knee-extension to place it on the ground. The peroneal muscles are also likely to lose their nerve supply, so there will also be inversion of the foot, while the front of the leg and the dorsum of the foot will lose sensory supply.

Damage (or local irritation) to part of the sciatic nerve is common from lower lumbar bone or disc pathology, most likely as root lesions. Total damage to the nerve is much more unusual, due to posterior wounds or posterior fractures and dislocations around the hip joint. This would lead to paralysis of the hamstrings and loss of all the muscles below the knee, together with a similar area of sensory loss, except for the medial side of the leg.

Injections are commonly given into the legs, most usually the buttocks and outer thigh. The latter has no major nerves to be damaged in the region below the greater trochanter and is a good site for personal injection, such as insulin for diabetics.

The region of the buttocks is less easy and in far too many cases the sciatic nerve has been damaged or even destroyed by injections. Injections limited to the upper and outer quadrant of the buttock should be safe but, even with this knowledge, damage has been done. The best advice is to make the injection a little below the iliac crest and behind the anterior superior iliac spine, or above and anterior to a line joining the tip of the greater trochanter and the posterior superior iliac spine (**Figure 252**).

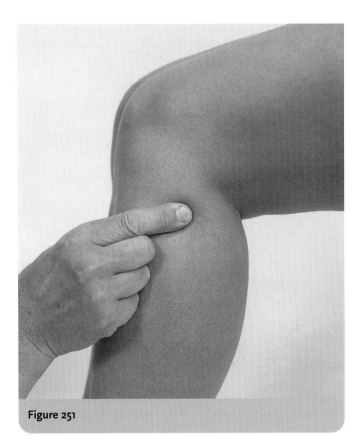

Figure 251

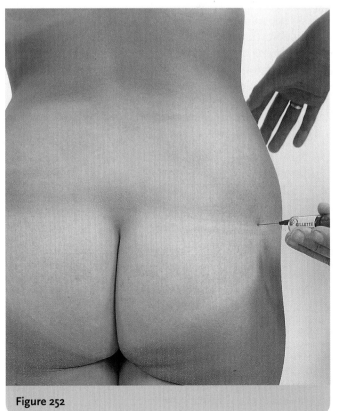

Figure 252

THE ARTERIES OF THE LEG

The femoral artery, the main axial artery to the leg, is a continuation of the external iliac, entering the leg at the mid-inguinal point (i.e. midway between the symphysis pubis and the anterior superior iliac spine; see page 96), becoming superficial in the femoral triangle in the upper ⅓ of the thigh (**Figure 253**). Being superficial, it, and the femoral vein to its medial side, are **vulnerable to injury**. It is also **available for cannulation** for a variety of clinical activities, e.g. renal angiography. From the femoral triangle it runs into the subsartorial canal, winds around the medial side of the femur under adductor magnus, to enter the popliteal fossa. If the leg is flexed and rotated slightly laterally at the hip, a line drawn from the mid-inguinal point to the adductor tubercle gives the surface projection in the upper ⅔ of the thigh.

In the popliteal fossa, now the **popliteal artery**, it lies deeply. If the knee is flexed, the tension of the fascia over the popliteal fossa is relaxed and the artery can be felt pulsating against the back of the tibial table, where it can also be **compressed in arterial bleeding (Figure 254)**. The femoral artery can also be compressed in the groin, over the head of the femur, or against the medial aspect of the femur in mid-thigh.

About level with the tibial tubercle, the popliteal artery divides into posterior and anterior tibial branches.

The posterior tibial artery runs down the leg with the tibial nerve, deep to gastrocnemius and soleus, to appear more superficially behind the medial side of the tibia. At the medial malleolus it lies about midway between the malleolus and the tendo calcaneus (with the nerve behind and lateral), before curving to the sustentaculum tali. Behind the malleolus the **pulsations should be felt** quite easily by light pressure against the lower part of the tibia, where it is also available for **compression in arterial bleeding (Figure 255)**. The order of structures from the medial malleolus laterally is tibialis posterior, flexor digitorum longus, posterior tibial artery (with its venae commitantes), tibial nerve and flexor hallucis longus; the last initially under the tendo calcaneus. From the ankle the posterior tibial artery runs into the sole of the foot, dividing into medial and lateral plantar arteries.

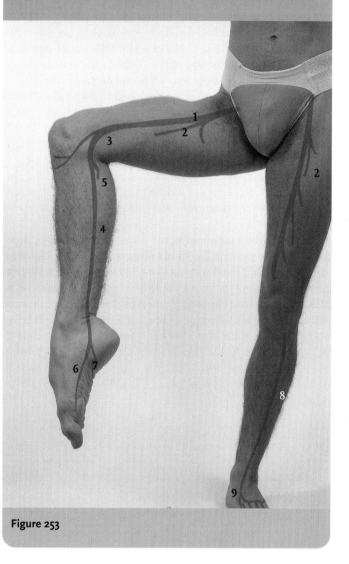

1 Femoral	6 Medial plantar
2 Profunda	7 Lateral plantar
3 Popliteal	8 Anterior tibial
4 Posterior tibial	9 Dorsalis pedis
5 Peroneal	

Figure 253

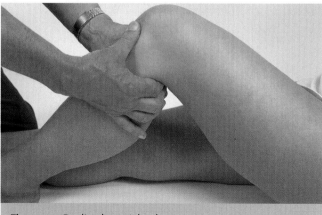

Figure 254 Popliteal arterial pulse.

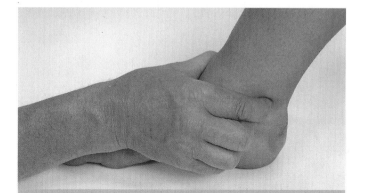

Figure 255 If there is difficulty in feeling the artery in the natural position, it can be helped by dorsiflexing and everting the foot.

The anterior tibial artery passes through the interosseous membrane into the front of the leg and then runs down on the membrane, towards the ankle, to lie on the front of the tibia. In the upper part of the leg it lies about midway between the tibial tubercle and the neck of the fibula, while at the ankle it is midway between the two malleoli. Passing into the foot, it runs lateral to the tendon of extensor hallucis longus, as the **dorsalis pedis artery**, before going through the space between the first and second metatarsals. The artery can be felt pulsating just lateral to the tendon of flexor hallucis longus, over the cuneiform bones and lateral to the base of the first metatarsal (**Figure 256**).

Palpation of the arterial pulses in the leg is often important clinically; they are frequently involved in changes in their walls, with consequent reduction in blood flow.

Although for routine **arterial cannulation** the radial artery is the most used, the dorsalis pedis is an excellent and safe alternative.

As the skin of the dorsum of the foot is of good quality with an axial blood supply through the dorsalis pedis vessels, it makes an excellent **free graft** based on the anterior tibial vessels, to which the accompanying nerve can be incorporated, if a suitable nerve is available in the recipient area, in addition to blood vessels.

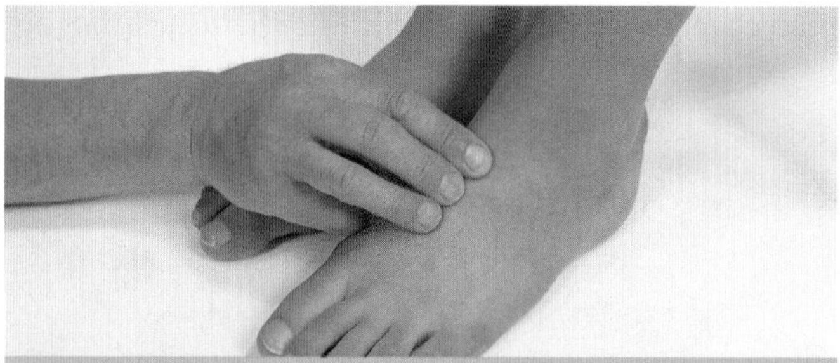

THE VEINS OF THE LEG

The veins in the leg are of particular clinical importance for a variety of reasons besides carrying the blood against gravity towards the heart. Stasis in the deep veins—from a variety of causes—commonly leads to thrombosis, which not only blocks the veins but may also lead to thrombi going into the circulation, ending most commonly, and often fatally, in the lungs. The superficial veins frequently become varicosed, with resultant deficiencies in superficial venous return.

The superficial venous drainage from the toes develops on the dorsum and, with veins from between the metatarsals, forms a dorsal venous arch.

The small (short) saphenous vein starts from the lateral aspect of the dorsal venous arch, and runs behind the lateral malleolus, up the back of the calf to the midline over the popliteal fossa. Here it pierces the popliteal fascia to join the popliteal vein (**Figure 257**).

The great (long) saphenous vein begins on the medial side of the dorsum of the foot from the venous arch. It runs up in front of the medial malleolus and then behind the medial condyles of the tibia and femur, before ascending superficially to the groin, initially along the posterior border of sartorius (**Figure 258**). It then passes through the deep fascia, via the saphenous opening, to join the femoral vein. The opening lies 3–4 cm below the inguinal crease, to the medial side of the

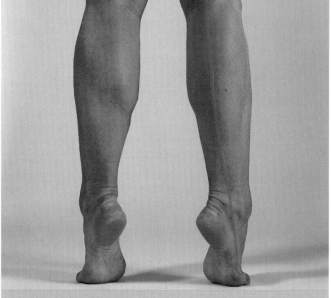

Figure 256 Dorsalis pedis pulse.

Figure 257 Small (short) saphenous vein.

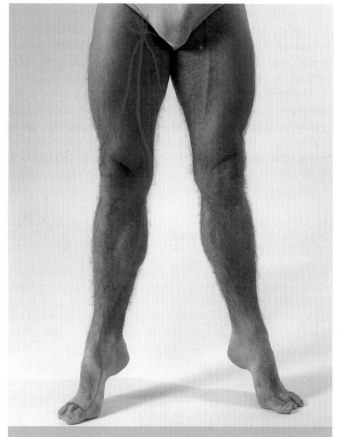

Figure 258 The great (long) saphenous vein.

femoral artery. Before passing deep, the vein is joined by a 'cartwheel' of veins, of which the most important are the **superficial external pudendal** from the genital region, the **superficial epigastric** from the lower abdominal wall, and the **superficial circumflex iliac**. Other veins join from the thigh, while linkages between the two saphenous veins are common, particularly below the knee. **Accessory saphenous veins** may also run into the great saphenous vein.

Both **saphenous veins have valves** to prevent the blood dropping downwards. They are also variably connected by several perforating and communicating veins with the deep veins, these also having valves to prevent blood returning to the superficial system. Valve failure is a feature of, and probably the most important cause of, varicose veins. Varicosities result in poor venous return from the superficial tissues of the leg with, in severe cases, ulceration.

The superficial veins in the foot offer an excellent **site for infusions** when they are visible and therefore readily accessible. If, however, they are small, contracted or hidden in fat or oedema, it may be necessary to cut down onto the great or, sometimes, the small saphenous vein at the ankle. Therefore knowledge of their positions is vital, so that accurate placing of the incision is made. The saphenous nerve runs with the great saphenous vein and this should be remembered, to avoid cutting the nerve, with the risk of developing a painful neuroma.

Because the main venous pump to the heart comes from the muscles (particularly soleus) acting on the deep veins, the superficial veins can often be discarded, and may have to be when they become severely varicosed and incompetent. They are also available as **vascular grafts** to replace arteries; most commonly for replacement of coronary arteries in cardiac bypass surgery. The whole of the great saphenous vein may be used for this purpose.

The deep veins follow the arteries, initially as venae commitantes, becoming popliteal to femoral veins. The femoral vein runs up medial to the artery in the femoral triangle, passing through the intermediate space of the femoral sheath, to become the external iliac vein (see page 96). In the femoral sheath it lies immediately lateral to the femoral canal, where care is needed to avoid perforation in femoral-hernial repair.

LYMPHATICS OF THE LEG

The main drainage from the foot runs onto the dorsum and thence along with the great saphenous vein. Those from the lateral side follow the small saphenous vein, to the popliteal fossa, where several lymph glands lie in the fat. Vessels then run deep, following the artery, to deep inguinal lymph nodes along the femoral vessels; some lymphatics may also run superficially, joining those following the great saphenous vein.

The lymphatics running with the great saphenous vein follow it to the inguinal region to end in superficial inguinal lymph nodes. **The superficial inguinal lymph nodes** compose a T-shaped group, receiving lymph from the area of vascular drainage of the great saphenous vein and its tributaries. The

transversely running group lies parallel to and below the inguinal ligament. The more lateral ones drain the superficial iliac region and the lower abdominal wall, and the more medial ones, the external genital region and the anus. The vertical group, lying along the saphenous vein, receive the superficial, and then deep drainage from the whole of the leg, except for those that have gone through the popliteal nodes (**Figure 258**).

Infections etc. from the lateral toes and side of the foot, together with the lateral part of the lower leg, may produce a response in the popliteal nodes. Being embedded in fat, these are less easy to feel than the inguinal nodes. The superficial inguinal lymph nodes drain a large area of the leg, and also the lower abdominal wall and the perineum. Lying in the hollow of the groin, they can easily be felt, often being palpable in the normal state (**Figure 259**). Pain and swelling in these nodes may indicate infection or malignancy in any part of their drainage. However, as they drain the perineum and anus, the latter being an infected region, reaction in these nodes is more likely to come from that source than from the leg.

From the superficial inguinal lymph nodes, vessels pass through the cribriform fascia to deep nodes on the femoral vessels and then through the femoral canal, which contains a lymph node, to the iliac nodes. Superficial drainage from the buttock follows the course of the leg or perineum, but the deeper ones run direct to the iliac lymph nodes.

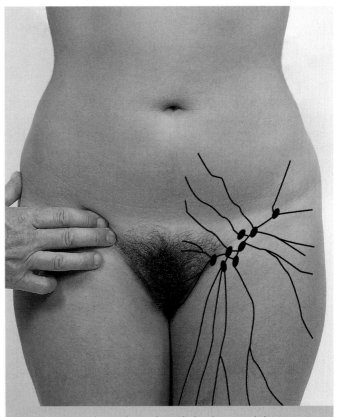

Figure 259 Lymphatic channels and glands around the groin.

Index